History of Ophthalmology 2

Academiae Ophthalmologicae Internationalis

History of Ophthalmology 2

Sub auspiciis
Academiae Ophthalmologicae Internationalis

Editor H.E. HENKES
Geervliet, The Netherlands
Associate Editor Cl. ZRENNER
Munich, F.R.G.

Kluwer Academic Publishers
Dordrecht / Boston / London

ISBN 0-7923-0273-7

Published by Kluwer Academic Publishers,
P.O. Box 17, 3300 AA Dordrecht, The Netherlands

Kluwer Academic Publishers incorporates the publishing programmes of D. Reidel, Martinus Nijhoff, Dr W. Junk and MTP Press.

Sold and distributed in the U.S.A. and Canada
by Kluwer Academic Publishers,
101 Philip Drive, Norwell, MA 02061, U.S.A.

In all other countries, sold and distributed
by Kluwer Academic Publishers Group,
P.O. Box 322, 3300 AH Dordrecht, The Netherlands

Reprinted from *Documenta Ophthalmologica*, Vol. 71, No. 2 (1989).

Printed in the Netherlands
printed on acid free paper

Documenta Ophthalmologica 71: 93–111, 1989.

Quantitative visual psychophysics during the period of European enlightenment. The studies of the astronomer and mathematician Tobias Mayer (1723–1762) on visual acuity and colour perception

O.-J. GRÜSSER
Department of Physiology, Freie Universität Berlin, Arnimallee 22, D-1000 Berlin 33

Introduction

In 1860 Gustav Theodor Fechner defined psychophysics as the "exact science of the relationship between body and mind". To realize this goal Fechner used and extended the measurements of psychophysical difference-thresholds by E.H. Weber and others who had observed that within certain limits the difference-threshold for a "just noticeable perceptual difference" E depended on stimulus intensity I_1, whereby the increase in I_1 to I_2 ($=\Delta I$) related to I_1 remained constant within certain limits of I_1 (cf. Wundt, 1893):

$$\Delta E \cong \frac{I_2 - I_1}{I_1} = \frac{\Delta I}{I_1} = \text{const.} \tag{1}$$

G.Th. Fechner called eq. (1) Weber's rule and generalized it in the following manner:

$$\Delta E \cong \frac{a\Delta I}{I} \text{[units of sensation]} = \text{const.} \tag{2}$$

The constant a of eq. (2) depends, of course, on the chosen units of sensation. The symbol $\cong$ in eqs. (1) and (2) does not mean mathematical identity but identity of sensation. The Belgian physiologist and physicist Plateau, who became interested in quantitative psychophysical studies, argued against Fechner's expression of Weber's rule, that the increase in sensation ΔE does not exist per se but is always related to a sensation E_1 caused by the stimulus I_1. Consequently, Plateau (1872, 1873) proposed another expression of Weber's rule:

$$\frac{\Delta E}{E} \cong a\frac{\Delta I}{I} \text{ [units of sensation]} \qquad (3)$$

Fechner derived his "psychophysical law" by integrating eq. (2) on both sides. The result was the well known "logarithmic" psychophysical rule, frequently called the Weber-Fechner law:

$$E \cong a \log I + b \text{ [units of sensation]} \qquad (4)$$

Plateau performed the same operation with eq. (4), which yields

$$\log E = a^{*} \log I + b^{*} \qquad (5)$$

and derived from this result the "psychophysical power law"

$$E = c.I^{\alpha} \text{ [units of sensation]} \qquad (6)$$

More recently the validity of this psychophysical power law has been investigated in particular by the American psychologist S.S. Stevens of the Harvard University and his coworkers (e.g. Stevens, 1951, 1957). Nowadays eq. (6) is often called "Steven's law".

In 1874 Ewald Hering, who was dissatisfied with the logarithmic law of Fechner as well as the power law of Plateau, proposed another relationship between E and I, derived from his general considerations on the interaction of the processes "assimilation" and "dissimilation" in neuronal networks (today called excitation and inhibition). For the perception of brightness and darkness he assumed a dissimilatory process W (white) and an assimilatory process S and demonstrated that the equation

$$E \cong \frac{W}{S + W} \text{ [units of sensation]} \qquad (7)$$

described the experimental data on brightness perception much better than Fechner's or Plateau's laws (Hering 1874, 1920).

Hering's law can be generally written as

$$E \cong \frac{aI}{1 + kI} \text{ [units of sensation]} \qquad (8)$$

This hyperbolic function gives the well-known S-shaped curve when E is plotted as a function of log I.

In several textbooks of modern physiology it is claimed that Weber and Fechner were the first to investigate the quantitative relationship between E and I. Handwerker, for example (in Schmidt/Thews, 1987), wrote that in 1850 G.Th. Fechner had introduced "the first useful technique by which the subjective sensation could be quantitatively described" and that his research had led to the "first psychophysical law by which the quantitative relationship between the dimension of physical intensity (I) and the subjective dimension of the strength of sensation (E)" was described.

The present study will argue that precise quantitative measurements on visual thresholds and the corresponding formulation of the psychophysical power law had been performed for the relationship between visual acuity and stimulus luminance 100 years before Fechner and 120 years before Plateau. This work, unknown to most modern sensory physiologists, but still mentioned by Hueck (1840), Weber (1852), Helmholtz (1866) and König (1897), was undertaken by the astronomer and mathematician Tobias Mayer (1723–1762) who in 1750 was appointed Professor of Applied Mathematics at the University of Göttingen, where he taught until his death in 1762. Mayer's studies in psychophysics also included the development of the first "metrical" colour space. His interest in visual psychophysics originated directly from practical problems arising in his work as an astronomer and cartographer. Mayer performed his investigations in the spirit of enlightenment, following the typical belief of many enlightened scientists of his time, derived from the success of physical mechanics, that quantitative studies are an important and meaningful way to understand nature.

Despite his being one of the most famous astronomers of his time, Mayer's early death was responsible for many of his scientific discoveries remaining unpublished and later forgotten. Some of his scientific papers were edited by the Göttingen professor of physics, Georg Christoph Lichtenberg (1742–1799), who carried out this work by order of King George III of England, at that time also the sovereign of the duchy of Hannover. Many of Mayer's scientific papers were first translated and published in 1972 by E.G. Forbes. His work on visual acuity, printed in Latin in 1752, was recently translated into English by Scheerer (1987). Since the majority of readers are most likely unacquainted with Mayer's biography, I will present a short outline before going on to describe his work in the two fields of visual psychophysics mentioned.

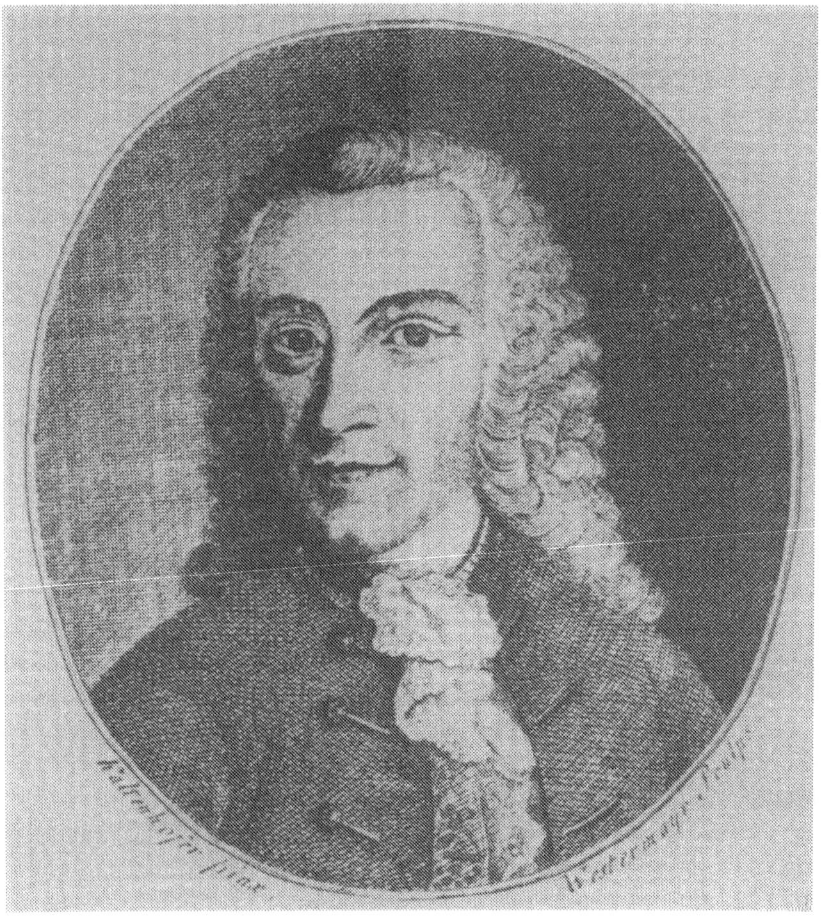

Fig. 1. Portrait of Tobias Mayer. Copper engraving by Kaltenhofer and Westermayer (from Zach, F.X. von (ed.): Allgemeine geographische Ephemeriden 3, Gotha, 1801, republished Roth/Bernhardt 1985).

Tobias Mayer (1723–1762)

Tobias Mayer (Fig. 1) descended from a family of craftsmen in the "Freie Reichstadt" Esslingen am Neckar, located in southern Germany (now Baden-Württemberg). He was born in 1723 in Marbach a.N., where the modest home of his family now serves as a small museum in his honour. His family returned to Esslingen a.N. in 1724 where his father was appointed "Brunnenmacher" of the city. He was a skillful craftsman and engineer and from him Tobias learned to draw and write before entering elementary school. Tobias was considered a child prodigee. As a school boy he drew many systematic maps of the city. A few of his remarkable watercolours of prospects from his home city have been preserved since his school days and are the only existing documents of buildings now vanished. Tobias's father died in 1730. Since Tobias had demonstrated brilliant intellectual ability, the city council decided to support his education with a fellowship and he was accepted into the "Alumnat" of the city, continuing his education in the old Latin school at Esslingen a.N., where he studied in Latin, Greek, religion, logic, history, rhetoric and geography (Kästner, 1763; Benzenberg, 1812; Eberhardt, 1924; Kommerell, 1941; Neumann, 1983; Roth and Bernhardt, 1985). In addition, at the expense of the city council, he was given private lessons by the "Constabler" G. Geiger in geometry, planimetry, construction of military buildings and mathematics applied to problems of the artillery. He was also supported by the shoemaker Kandler (1712–1771), who had a deep interest in algebra and geometry, and was considered a bit of a character by his townsmen. Mayer wrote about Kandler "my shoemaker and I did fit very well together, since he loved mathematical sciences and had money to buy the books, but no time to read them, since he had to make shoes. I, however, had time to read, but no money to buy books. Thus he bought the books which I wanted to read and I instructed him in the evening when he had finished his daily duties, on all those items which I found noticeable in the books . . . ." (Benzenberg, 1812).

As a fellow of the "Alumnat" Mayer also had to teach younger pupils. These educational duties, along with his mathematical prowess, led to Mayer's first book published at the age of 18, when he was still a pupil in the upper class of the Latin School ("Lyceum"): "Neue und allgemeine Art, alle Aufgaben aus der Geometrie vermittelst der geometrischen Linien leicht aufzulösen. Insbesonders wie alle regulären und irregulären Vielecke, davon ein Verhältnis ihrer Seiten gegeben, in den Circul geometrisch sollen eingeschrieben werden, samt einer kurzen hier zu nötigen Buchstaben-Rechenkunst und Geometrie. Als Erstlinge ans Licht gestellt von Tobias Mayer" (1741). The book deals with basic and general algebra, rules for solving algebraic equations of second and third order and general rules of geometry.

In 1743 Mayer moved to Augsburg, where his elder half-brother, Georg Wilhelm Mayer, worked as a craftsman. Tobias Mayer presumably worked in Augsburg as a "Kupferstecher" and "Schriftstecher" and used his free time to write his second book on mathematics "Mathematischer Atlas" (1745). This work indicated that he had acquired in the meantime a good knowledge of astronomy and geography. Like his first work, the second book also dealt primarily with applied mathematics. In 1746 he moved to Nürnberg where he was hired by the publishing company Homann-Erben, reknowned for their maps. Meanwhile, Mayer had become widely known for his precise cartographic knowledge and abilities. In Nürnberg he initiated improvements in map production and became interested in the techniques for an exact astronomical determination of the geographic position longitudes, lattitudes of German cities. He was not satisfied with the precision of the astronomical knowledge of his time and thought to improve the computation of the moon – and star tables. In addition, he performed systematic observations at the astronomical observatory in Nürnberg. He published many articles on cartography and astronomy (Forbes 1980, Roth and Bernhard 1985) and became famous in these fields. Despite having never attended university, in 1750 he was offered a chair as Professor of Economy (Applied Mathematics) at the University of Göttingen, which had been founded in 1737. Mayer moved from Nürnberg to Göttingen and developed there an extensive research and teaching program. Soon he became director of the Göttingen observatory, where he continued his astronomical observations. He produced precise maps of the moon, extended the tables of stellar positions, and improved the astronomical observation techniques for measuring the geographic locations of any spot on the globe. During the 18th century the determination of the geographic position of vessels at sea was still rather imprecise and vague. This situation led in 1714 to the establishment of a "Board of Longitude" by the British Parliament, which offered a prize for new and reliable methods of determining one's position at sea. In general, there were two solutions to this problem: The construction of precise clocks and the use of an "astronomical clock" by the development of exact tables for the position of the moon, sun and selected stars in the sky. Tobias Mayer naturally chose the second approach and developed in 1753 the basis for the determination of geographic longitude at sea. Supported by the famous mathematician Leonhard Euler (1707–1783), Mayer submitted his results to the British Parliament in order to receive the afore-mentioned gratification from the "Board of Longitude". After a rather long delay caused in part by the Seven Years War (1756–1763) Tobias Mayer was awarded the money posthumously, but instead of the 10,000 Pounds promised, his widow received only 3,000 which was nonetheless an enormous sum at that time.

In his everyday work with astronomical instruments, Tobias Mayer was confronted with the problem of visual acuity and the dependence of visual resolution on illumination. He had developed several technical innovations for reading off the angles on his astronomical instruments (e.g. special micrometers) and tried to enhance the precision of these instruments by repeating the reading of the observational values and computing algebraic means. This method with which every scientist today is familiar, was new in

Mayer's time. While developing a theory of measurement error, he also encountered the problem of visual acuity, which he decided to measure in the human observer. In the Latin publication of his results "Experimenta circa visus aciem" (Mayer 1755), it is interesting that he justified his measurements by two arguments: the insufficient science of errors and the limited knowledge of the "most important source of errors", namely "the weakness of the human senses". Mayer did not ask whether it is at all possible to measure psychophysical threshold and to deduce quantitative rules from these measurements. This problem, he considered a priori as the "natural" way for a scientist to solve practical problems.

The same attitude was also present in Mayer's second psychophysical investigation "De affinitate colorum" (1758). Again it was a practical question which led to this research, namely the colouring of his maps. He was not satisfied by the rather variable outcome when different colours were used. In the course of his study of subtractive colour mixtures he developed an early trichromatic theory of colour vision. Thomas Young (1773–1829), who studied at the University of Göttingen in 1793 and collaborated with G.Ch. Lichtenberg, became acquainted with the colour space of Tobias Mayer and his model of subtractive colour mixture. Lichtenberg published Mayer's manuscript on colour studies in 1775 ("Opera inedita Tobiae Mayeri I", Göttingen, p. 93–103).

The two psychophysical publications of Mayer were side products of an extremely creative scientist who remained active in astronomy up until his death in 1762, a result of influenza acquired during the occupation of the city of Göttingen by French troops during the Seven Years War. Tobias Mayer was well-known during his lifetime as one of the leading astronomers, as an ingenious cartographer, inventor of mechanical instruments and as a scientist who successfully applied mathematics and mechanics to many problems in the natural sciences. The list of courses and academic lectures which he delivered during his ten years as professor at the University of Göttingen is remarkable and comprises practical geometry, algebra, astronomy, construction and use of machines, civil architecture, military architecture, pyrotechniques, fortification and ballistics, optics, including dioptrics and catoptrics, mathematical geography, cartography, spherical trigonometry, the use and construction of astronomical instruments and "precepts of the art of drawing and developing mathematical constructions" (Forbes, 1980).

Mayer's measurements on the dependence of visual acuity on the illumination of the stimulus pattern

The precision of astronomical measurements had, of course, improved with the introduction of the telescope by Galileo Galilei (1611), but was limited nonetheless not only by the instruments available (e.g. telescopic astrolabes quadrants etc.), but also by the visual acuity of the observers. The classification of stars according to their brightness into six classes by the Greek astronomer Hipparchos had been introduced about 150 B.C. and the astronomers knew that the precision of astronomical readings depended on the brightness category of a star. Hipparch's classification was used up until the 19th century when photometric measurements of the light received from a given star became feasible. Then it was found that the six brightness classes corresponded metrically to the logarithm of light intensity measured by the photometer (Stevens, 1957). During the time of Tobias Mayer, this relationship was unknown, but he realized in the course of his observations that the measurements of the astronomical coordinates of a bright star were much more exact than those of a dimmer one. To improve the reading of astronomical or physical instruments he suggested using the algebraic mean of many measurements instead of single reading. Mayer also became aware that the outcome depended on the illumination of the scales. Apparently he did not know that the English astronomer and physicist, Robert Hooke (1635–1703), the "Curator of Experiments" of the Royal Society in London, had demonstrated as early as 1674 at a Royal Society meeting that visual acuity could be measured by means of black and white gratings. The report on Hooke's demonstration was published by Birch in 1756. "Mr Hooke made an experiment with the ruler divided into such parts as being placed at certain distance from the eye, appeared to subtend a minute of a degree; and being earnestly and curiously viewed by all persons present, it appeared, that not any person, being present, being placed at the assigned distance, was able to distinguish those parts which appeared at the bigness of a minute, but that they appeared confuse". Hooke speculated that visual acuity is a result of the "diameter of the optic nerve fibers forming the inner layer of the retina" (Hooke 1705, p. 98). Many attentive observers had, of course, noted the qualitative dependence of visual acuity on the strength of illumination. This was mentioned, for example, by George Berkeley (1684–1753) in his "An Essay towards a new Theory of Vision" (1709, Sect. LIV) and by Christian Wolff (1679–1754), who noted that visual acuity decreased from the center towards the periphery of the visual field. Like Hooke, Wolff assumed that under optimal conditions of illumination the *minimum visibile* is related in a 1:1 fashion to the density of the "optic fibers" in the retina

(Wolff, 1725, p. 381–382). Wolff also discussed a general rule, not only for the eye but also for the skin, on the relation between sensory resolution and density of innervation. Since Wolff's publications were generally known by the German scientists of his time and Tobias Mayer recommended the use of Wolff's books for his lectures, it seems fairly likely that he was acquainted with Wolff's remarks on the general relationship of visual acuity and strength of illumination.

Tobias Mayer reported on his experimental data and conclusions at a session of the "Societas Regiae Scientiarium" in Göttingen on April 6th, 1754 and published his data one year later in the journal of the society ("Commentarii Societatis Regiae Scientiarium Gottingensis. Tomus IV)

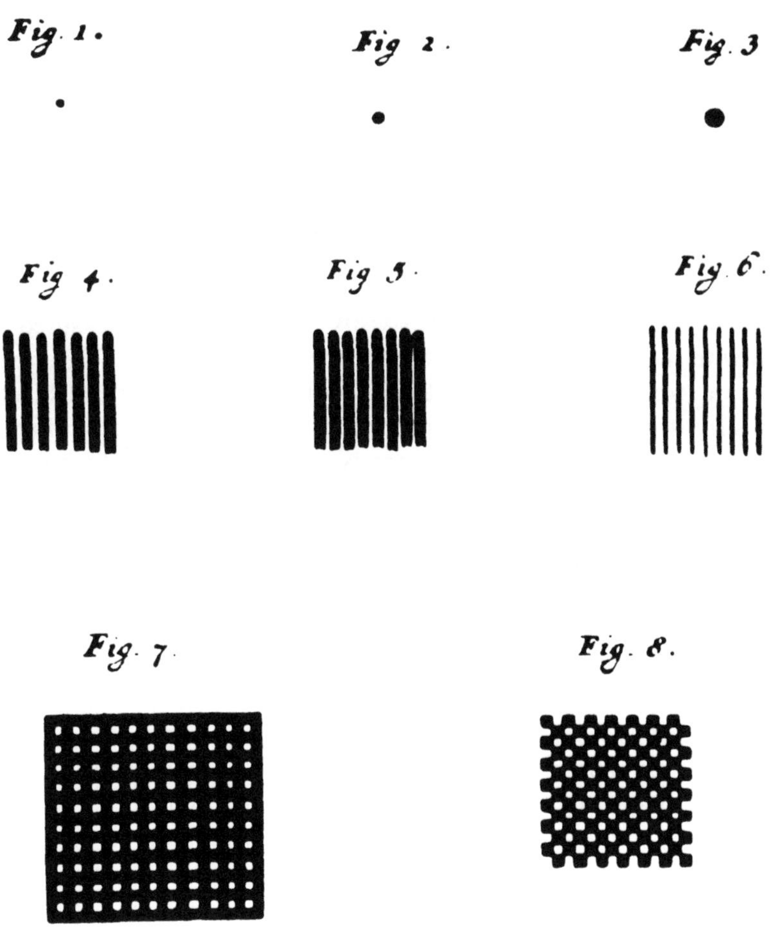

Fig. 2. Stimulus patterns used in the experiments of Tobias Mayer (1755). For further explanations see text.

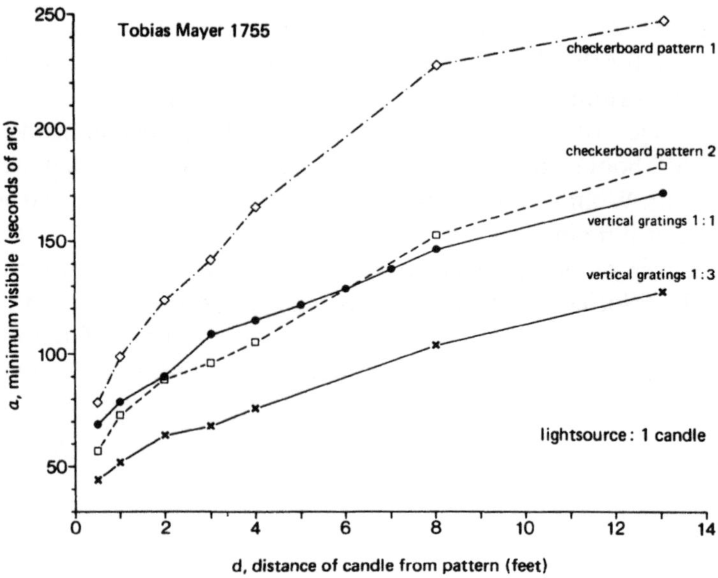

Fig. 3. Relationship of the minimum visibile, the minimum angle α of resolution (ordinate) and the distance d of the light source, a candle, from the stimulus pattern used to determine visual acuity. Data given in Mayers publication (1755) are plotted in linear coordinates.

under the title "Experimenta circa visus aciem". Mayer measured visual acuity with two different classes of visual stimuli: black dots of different sizes placed on white paper, and patterned stimuli, namely vertical black and white stripes with equal or unequal white and black periods and checkerboard patterns (Fig. 2). In his first series of experiments he illuminated the patterns uniformly by daylight and determined the distance required by his subjects to see the dots or discriminate the gratings or checkerboard patterns from a homogeneous grey. He wrote that if he "removed [the patterns] somewhat more, the whole pattern was estimated to have the same quasi grey colour". He concluded that on measuring the visual acuity with the first type, a black dot on a white background was just recognizable when its diameter was related to the distance d by 1/6000, which corresponds to a value of about 34 seconds of arc. When he brought the stimulus pattern into very bright sunlight, he observed a reduction in visual acuity, which he correctly explained by the effects of blinding and straylight in the eye. The "visual acuity of the second type", determined by gratings or checkerboard patterns, was considered by Mayer as the "real" visual acuity, since with this method the perception of visual structures would be used as a criteron. For the grating "Fig. 4" in Fig. 2 he found a minimum visibile of 47 seconds of arc and for the other patterns Figs. 5–8, threshold values of 60, 30, 40 and 62 seconds of arc when they were illuminated by moderate daylight.

After repeated observations he was convinced that measurements of visual acuity with the gratings and checkerboard pattern were reliable and he began a second set of psychophysical experiments to determine the dependence of the minimum visibile on the illumination strength of the stimulus patterns. He used a candle for these measurements and varied the distance d of the candle from the stimulus pattern. For the relationship of the minimum visibile α and the distance d he found the following rules:

$$\alpha \;=\; k \cdot d^{1/3} \text{ [seconds of arc]} \tag{9}$$

whereby the constant k was 79 for the grating with equal black and white stripes, 52 for the gratings with unequal black and white stripes, 73 and 99 for the checkerboard pattern; d was measured in feet. He presented the results of his experiments, which he performed "at night" with the "direct light of a tallow candle", in several tables. In Fig. 3 Mayer's data are plotted on linear coordinates.

Since the illumination intensity I of the stimulus pattern decreases with the square of the distance d between light source and visual pattern, Mayer deduced from eq. (9) a general relationship between the minimum visibile α and the luminance I of the stimulus pattern and its background (black-white contrast was constant):

$$\alpha \;=\; k \cdot I^{-1/6} \text{ [seconds of arc]} \tag{10}$$

Since the visual acuity V can be defined as the reciprocal value of the minimum visibile one can transform eq. (10) into

$$V \;=\; \frac{1}{\alpha} \;=\; k^* \cdot I^{1/6} \text{ [seconds of arc}^{-1}\text{]} \tag{11}$$

In Fig. 4 Mayer's data are plotted in a log-coordinate system including the power function of eq. (11) with the constants k* published by Mayer. It is evident from this figure that the relationship between empirical data and theory was remarkably well described by Mayer's power law.

Interestingly, Mayer immediately extended his psychophysical observations to another problem: He estimated the intensity of daylight relative to that of the candles applied in his studies by measuring visual acuity and extrapolating eq. (11). He concluded that moderate daylight corresponded to approximately 25 candles illuminating the stimulus pattern from one foot distance. When one reads the remarkably clear publication of Mayer, it is impressive to realize how obvious the application of mathematical rules to subjective sensations was for him. It is evident that the spirit of enlightenment and the success of mechanical physics facilitated the scientific attitude

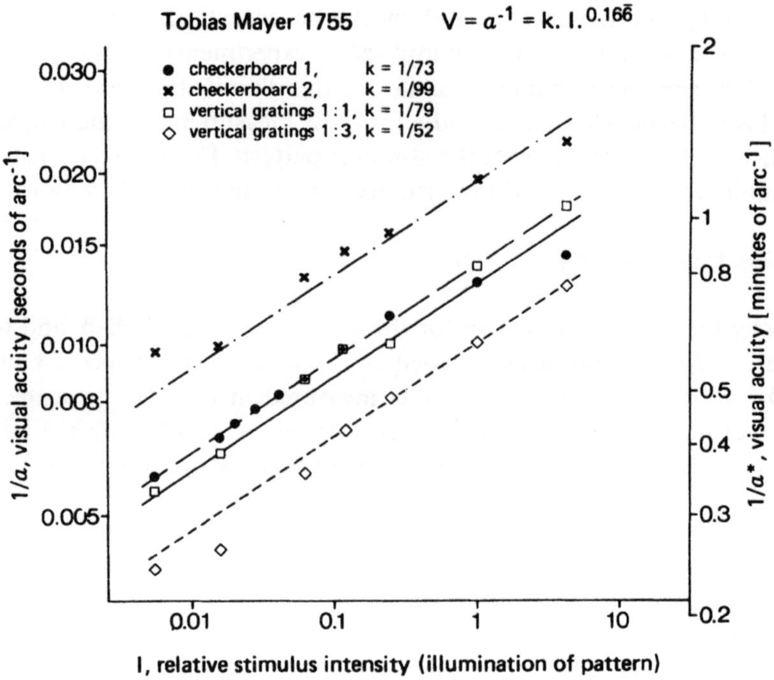

Fig. 4. Relationship of the visual acuity (ordinate) in seconds of arc (left side) or minutes of arc (right side) is plotted as a function of the illumination of the stimulus patterm. Data from Mayer 1755 are plotted in a logarithmic coordinate system. The straight lines correspond to the power functions described by Mayer for the respective data.

characteristic of Mayer's publications. The "L'homme machine" was published by J.O. LaMettrie (1709–1751) a few years before (1748) Mayer's study. This work characterizes very well the mechanical interpretation of biological functions in man and animals, a concept which had been favoured most prominently a century before Tobias Mayer by Descartes in his posthumously published work "Traité de l'homme" (1664, Latin version: "Tractatus de homine", 1662). On the other hand, Mayer's sober and pragmatic approach to solving scientific problems was likely influenced by his individual background, his descent from a family of successful craftsmen and his activities as a schoolboy.

Mayer's quantitative rules of subtractive colour mixture and his construction of a three-dimensional colour space

Mayer's studies on colour perception and his efforts to construct a "colour body" representing human colour perception were again triggered by practical problems. He struggled with the difficulties of the craftsmen in producing identical colours in multicolour maps, as the results frequently did not satisfy the expectations of the scientist who had plotted them. In 1757 Mayer taught a course at the University of Göttingen on "The drawing and colouring of geometrical diagrams, fortifications and architectonic schemes" (Forbes 1980). It is fairly probable that he developed his quantitative descriptions of the colour space in preparation for this course. At a meeting of the Royal Society of Sciences at Göttingen on November 18th, 1758, Mayer reported on his efforts to construct a "colour triangle" from the three "main colours" Red, Yellow and Blue, and adding White or Black to the colour mixtures he was led to the construction of a three-dimensional hexaedric colour space. His talk was reported in the "Göttingische Anzeigen von Gelehrten Sachen unter der Aufsicht der Königlichen Gesellschaft der Wissenschaften, 147. Stück, 9. Dezember 1758" Mayer summarized his studies on colour vision in a manuscript "De affinitate colorum commentatio", which was published by Lichtenberg with the note "lecta in conventu publico d. 18. Nov. 1758" in the "Opera inedita Tobiae Mayeri" in 1775. Mayer asked the question which and how many colour hues man can discriminate and whether a quantitative relationship can be found for this ability when the various hues were produced by mixing different pigments. In his experimental studies he mixed three elementary pigments (red, yellow, blue) according to the rules mentioned below. Thus Mayer studied systematically the rules of subtractive colour mixture. His investigation led, of course, to other colour mixture rules than those resulting from similar efforts using the technique of additive colour mixture, i.e. the summation of spectral colours as discussed by Newton in his studies (Newton, 1730). Mayer recognized the differences between subtractive and additive colour mixtures, as he mentioned that with Newton's method the mixture of three adequately chosen spectral colours gives "white", while with his method a "dark grey" was obtained. He was convinced, however, that three colours are sufficient to define colour space. This was mentioned by him in 1745 in his "Mathematischer Atlas", in which he chose red, yellow and blue as primitive colours, seen also in the rainbow or in the spectrum of sunlight produced by a prism, in addition to some "secondary", i.e. mixed colours.

In Mayer's studies the hue F of a colour mixture from 2 or 3 primary colour pigments depended, of course, on the relative amount of mixed pigments. Mayer chose the following rule:

$$\begin{aligned} F &= R^{n}\, Y^{m}\, B^{(12-n-m)} \\ n + m &= 12 \end{aligned} \qquad (12)$$

With this notation Mayer meant not exponentials but an addition of three colour pigments (red R, yellow Y, blue B). Today we would write his expression so:

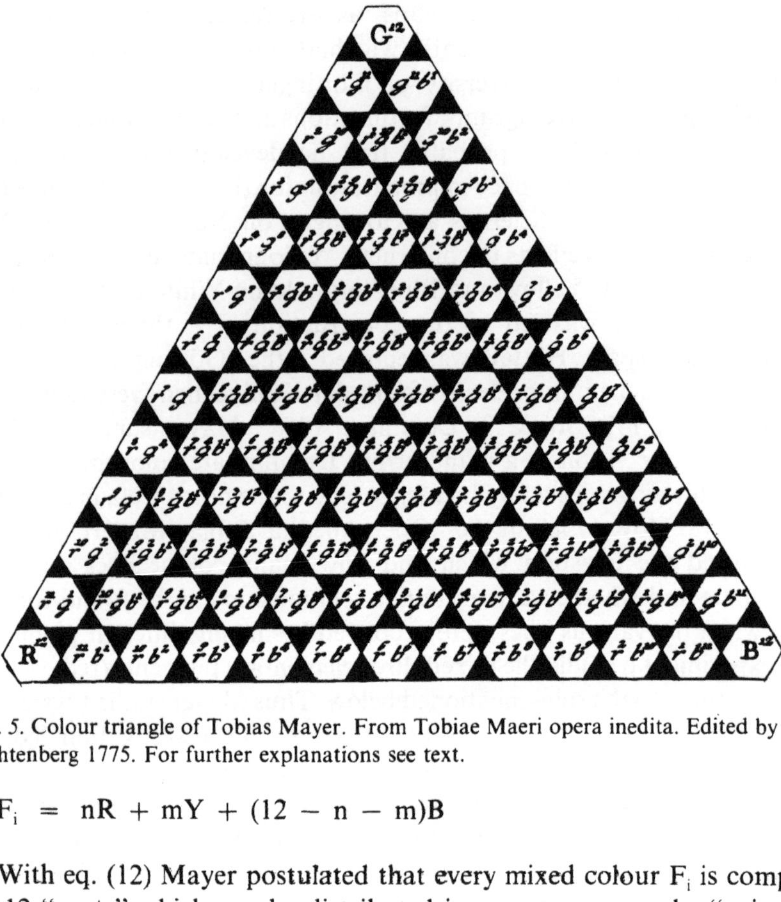

Fig. 5. Colour triangle of Tobias Mayer. From Tobiae Maeri opera inedita. Edited by G.Ch. Lichtenberg 1775. For further explanations see text.

$$F_i = nR + mY + (12 - n - m)B \tag{13}$$

With eq. (12) Mayer postulated that every mixed colour F_i is composed of 12 "parts" which can be distributed in any manner to the "primitive" colours red (R), yellow (Y) and blue (B). The neutral colour Grey received in Mayer's notation R^4 Y^4 B^4 and was placed in the center of his "colour triangle" .

Mayer deduced from eq. (12) a two-dimensional geometric representation of the "pure" mixed colours, an early version of the colour triangle (Fig. 5), but his colour plane was related to a subtractive colour mixture. Mayer's colour triangle consisted of the three elementary or "primitive" colours placed on the corners of the triangle, 23 colours mixed from 2 simple colours and 55 colours mixed from 3 simple colours. Thus Mayer's colour triangle was composed of 91 hues which can be easily distinguished by a human observer and are organized regularly in the plane of the triangle according to eq. (12).

Black and white were not considered as primary colours by Mayer but he knew, of course, that adding black or white pigments to a subtractive colour

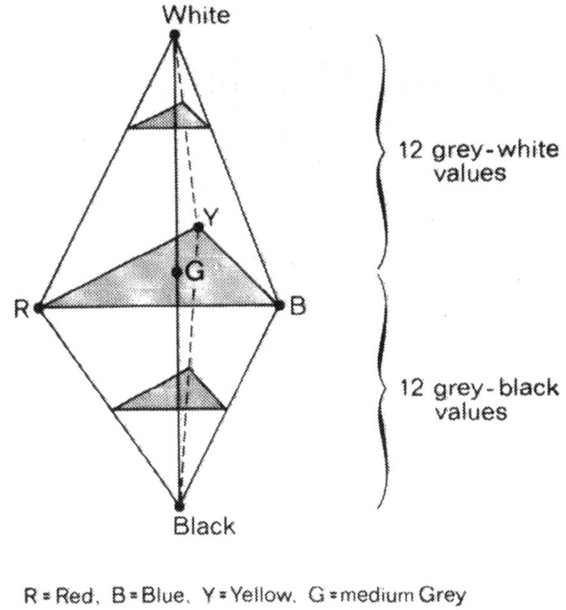

Fig. 6. Mayer's hexaedric colour space. The colour triangle of Fig. 5 forms the triangle separating the upper "light" and the lower "shadow" part of Mayer's hexaedric colour space.

mixture changed the chroma. He considered the addition of black and white as a way to change the "degree of light" or "degree of shadow" in a certain colour. To represent the white or black components in a colour he extended his colour triangle to a colour space, a hexaeder with a black-white axis placed orthogonally to the plane and through the center of the colour triangle. The tips of the hexaeder are "pure White" or "pure Black" (Fig. 6). Any colour, F_i, mixed with black or white could be attributed to one point in the colour hexaeder according to the following equations:

$$F_i = W^d R^a Y^b B^c \qquad (14)$$

for the "white half" of the hexaeder

and

$$F_i = S^e R^a Y^b B^c \qquad (15)$$

for the "shadow part" of the hexaeder.

The notation again corresponds to that of eq. (12) and $(a + b + c + d)$ or $(a + b + c + e) = 12$. Mayer illustrated his hexaedric colour space in tables and pointed out in his papers that the colour space is composed of 91 "perfect colours" (colores perfecti) corresponding to the colour triangle, 364 "pale colours (colores pallidi) in the light part of the colour space and 364 "dark colours" (colores obscuri) in the shadow part of the hexaeder. Thus Mayer's colour space consisted of 819 different positions corresponding to diverse hues, which in Mayer's opinion a human observer could easily distinguish. To illustrate this idea Mayer produced a wax model of his colour space out of 819 wax balls containing pigments according to the rules of subtractive colour mixture as mentioned above. For example, the second "layer" above the triangle of "perfect colours" has the general notation $W^2 R^m Y^n B^{(10-n-m)}$ and consists of 66 different hues.

Today the efforts of Tobias Mayer in constructing a colour space out of the results of subtractive colour mixture can be considered as a first step towards an experimentally supported theory of colour vision. It should be pointed out, however, that his interest was not primarily in colour vision but in the application of a metrically defined colour system, which facilitated the selection of colours for technical drawings, maps etc. Using the techniques of his time, Mayer attempted what was done later more precisely by Wilhelm Ostwald (1853–1927) and Munsell (Krantz 1972), namely to develop a metrically defined colour system with a specific position for each hue. In his equations Mayer assumed a linear operation of the 3 independent primaries. He realized of course that more than 819 colours could be mixed, having a place within the colour space (e.g. 1.5W + 2.5R + 5Y + 3B), but he claimed that a human observer could not discriminate this colour from its immediate neighbours in the colour space (e.g. 2W + 2R + 5Y + 3B).

Mayer's quantitative construction of a colour space, as his ideas and measurements on visual acuity, were not appreciated by the physiologists of his time. His approach to the formulation of psychophysical laws also came two generations too early. Sixty years later, J.W. Goethe studied the publications of Tobias Mayer while working on his anti-Newtonian colour theory. Goethe wrote in his "Materialien zur Geschichte der Farbenlehre" on Mayer: "Since he has an atomistic approach [in his scientific work] his treatment of colour vision is not at all sufficient", but he considered that in Mayer's work the "straitforward, sound, common sense" ("der gerade gesunde Menschenverstand") was evident (Goethe, 1810, p. 222).

Summary

During the sixth decade of the 18th century, Tobias Mayer, Professor of Astronomy and Applied Mathematics (Economy) at the University of

Göttingen, performed two investigations on quantitative visual psychophysics. He deduced a power law for the dependence of visual acuity on the intensity of light by which the stimulus pattern was illuminated. In his measurements he compared visual acuity determined with single black dots and visual acuity measured with gratings or checkerboard patterns; the latter he considered as the "real" measurement of visual acuity.

Mayer also developed a three-dimensional hexaedric colour space from the definition of subtractive colour mixtures of three primary pigments (red, yellow, blue). This colour space can be considered as the predecessor of the later colour tables of Ostwald and Munsell. Mayer gave a simple quantitative description of each of the 819 hues in his colour space.

Both psychophysical studies developed out of Mayer's interest in practical problems in astronomy and cartography. Mayer's main scientific merits were in the field of astronomy and mathematical geography. His psychophysical studies were performed in the spirit of enlightenment with the a priori assumption that the performance of the human perceptual machinery can be measured quantitatively and that the results are adequately expressed by mathematical rules. Mayer's achievements in the fields of mathematics, physics, astronomy and cartography were recently summarized by the extensive historical research of G.F. Forbes. In the present report a short biographical note precedes the description of Mayer's psychophysical studies.

Acknowledgements

The paper was written while the author was supported by an "Akademie-Stipendium" of the Stiftung Volkswagenwerk, Hannover. I thank Mrs. J. Dames and Dr. R. Kremer, Dept. of History, Dartmouth College, Hanover, NH, USA for their comments and assistance in the English translation of the manuscript.

References

Benzenberg JF. Erstlinge von Tobias Mayer aufs neue herausgegeben. Nebst einigen Nachrichten von seinen Erfindungen und seinem Leben. Düsseldorf: J.C. Schreiner, 1812.

Berkeley G. An essay towards a new theory of vision. Dublin: J. Pepyat 1709 In: Luce A.A, Jessop T.E, eds. Berkeley, G. Works, Vol. I, p 141–239. Edinburgh: Nelson, 1948.

Birch T. The history of the Royal Society of London. Vol. 3. London (repr. Johnson, New York 1968) 1756.

Descartes R. L'homme de René Descartes et un traitté de la formation du foetus (ed. L. de la Forge). Paris: Girard, 1664. German translation in Rothschuh KE. (1969: René Descartes "Über den Menschen (1632) sowie "Beschreibung des menschlichen Körpers" (1648) nach der ersten französischen Ausgabe übersetzt und mit einer historischen Einleitung und Anmerkung versehen. Heidelberg: Schneider 202 p.

Eberhardt P. Urkundliche Beiträge zur Jugendgeschichte des Astronomen Johann Tobias Mayer. In: Eberhardt P, ed. Aus Alt-Esslingen. Esslingen: O. Bechtle, 1924, 207–218.

Fechner GT. Elemente der Psychophysik. Vol. 1. Leipzig: Breitkopf und Härtel, 1860. Reprint: Amsterdam: Bonset 1964, 336 p.

Forbes EG. Tobias Mayer's Opera inedita, 1971. The first translation of the Lichtenberg edition of 1775. London: Macmillan.

Forbes EG. The Unpublished Writings of Tobias Mayer. 3 Vols. Göttingen: Vandenhoeck and Ruprecht, 1972.

Forbes, EG. Tobias Mayer (1723–62): Pioneer of Enlightened Science in Germany. Göttingen: Vandenhoeck and Ruprecht, 1980; 248 p.

Goethe JW. Materialien zur Geschichte der Farbenlehre. In: Goethes Naturwissenschaftliche Schriften, Hrsg. K. Goedeke, Vol. II. Stuttgart, Berlin: J.G. Cotta, 1910; 282 p.

Handwerker H. Allgemeine Sinnesphysiologie. In: Schmidt RF, Thews G, eds. Physiologie des Menschen. Berlin, Heidelberg: Springer, 1987; 186–206.

Helmholtz H von. Handbuch der physiologischen Optik, 1866. Hamburg, Leipzig: L. Voss, 2nd ed., 1896; 1334 p.

Hering E. Zur Lehre vom Lichtsinn. VI. Grundzüge einer Theorie des Farbensinnes. Ber k u k Akad Wiss, Wien, 1874; 70: 169.

Hering E. Grundzüge der Lehre vom Lichtsinn. Berlin: Springer, 1920; 294 p.

Hooke R. The Posthumous Works. London: Smith and Walford, 1705.

Hueck A. Über die Grenzen des Sehvermögens. Müllers Arch Anat Physiol wiss Med 1840; 82–97.

Kästner AG. Elogium Tobiae Mayeri, 1763. Göttingen (reprint: Marbach, 1984).

Kommerell V. Tobias Mayer. Mathematiker, Physiker, Astronom. In: Uhland R, ed. Schwäbische Lebensbilder, Vol. 2. Stuttgart: Kohlhammer, 1941; p. 351–66.

König A. Die Abhängigkeit der Sehschärfe von der Beleuchtungsintensität. Ber Königl Preuss Akad Wiss 1897; 559–75.

Krantz DH. Visual Scaling. In: Jameson D, Hurwich LM eds Visual Psychophysics, Vol VII/4 of Handbook of Sensory Physiology. Berlin, Heidelberg New York: Springer, 1972; 660–89.

LaMettrie JO. L'homme machine, 1751. Engl. transl. in: Bussey GC, ed. Man a machine. La Salle: Open Court, 1912; 216 p.

Lichtenberg G.Ch. Tobiae Mayeri. Opera inedita I. Göttingen: Vandenhoeck, 1775.

Mayer T. Neue und allgemeine Art, alle Aufgaben aus der Geometrie vermittelst der geometrischen Linien leichter aufzulösen; insbesondere wie alle reguläre und irreguläre Vielecke, davon ein Verhältnis ihrer Seiten gegeben in den Circul geometrisch sollen eingeschrieben werden, samt einer kurzen hierzu nötigen Buchstaben-Rechenkunst und Geometrie. Als Erstlinge an das Licht gestellet von Tobias Majern. Mathem Cult Esslingen, 1741.

Mayer T. Mathematischer Atlas, in welchem auf 60 Tabellen alle der Mathematik vorgestellt, und nicht allein überhaupt zu bequemer Wiederholung, sondern auch den Anfängern besonders zur Aufmunterung durch deutliche Beschreibung und Figuren entworfen werden, von Tobias Majern. Philomath Augsburg, 1745.

Mayer T. Experimente über die Schärfe des Gesichtssines. Göttinger Gelehrte Anzeigen Nr. 47. 20. April 1754; 401–402.

Mayer T. Experimenta circa visus aciem. Comment Soc Reg Sci Gottingensis 1755; 4: 97–112.

Mayer T. De affinitate colorum (Über die Verwandtschaft der Farben). Göttinger Gelehrte Anzeigen Nr. 147. 9. Dezember 1758; 1385–9.

Mayer T. De affinitate colorum commentations, 1758. In: Lichtenberg 1775.

Neumann F. Tobias Mayer – Leben und Werk. Marbach, 1983; 40 p.

Newton I. Opticks or a treatise of the reflections, refractions, inflections and colours of light, 1730. Reprint New York: Dover Edition, 4th edition, 1952; 406 p.

Plateau J. Sur la mesure des sensations physique, et sur la loi qui lie l'intensité de ces sensations à l'intensité de la cause excitante. Bull de l'Acad Roy Belg 1872; 33: 376–88.

Plateau J. Über die Messung physischer Empfindungen und das Gesetz, welches die Stärke dieser Empfindungen mit der Stärke der erregenden Ursache verknüpft. Poggendorfs Annalen der Physik und Chemie, 5. Reihe 1873; 30: 465–76.

Roth E. Tobias Meyer – ein beinahe vergessenes Genie. In Beiträge zur Landeskunde, Beilage zum Staatsanzeiger Baden-Württemberg Nr, 5, 1985; 1–6.

Roth E, Bernhardt W. Tobias Mayer 1723–1762. Vermesser des Meeres, der Erde und des Himmels, Esslingen a.N.: Stadtarchiv 1985, 182p.

Scheerer G. Tobias Mayer – Experiments on visual acuity. Spatial Vision 1987; 2: 81–97.

Stevens SS. Mathematics, measurement and psychophysics. In: Stevens, S.S. (ed) Handbook of experimental psychology. New York: Wiley, 1951; 1–49.

Stevens SS. The psychophysical law. Psychol Rev 1957; 64: 153–181.

Weber EH. Über den Raumsinn und die Empfindungskreise in der Haut und im Auge. Ber Königl Sächs Akad Wiss, Math-phys-Classe 1852; 85–164.

Wolff Ch. Vernünftige Gedancken vom Gebrauche der Theile in Menschen, Thieren und Pflantzen, den Liebhabern der Wahrheit mitgetheilet, 1725. Frankfurt/Leipzig: Renger. Reprint Hildesheim: G. Olms 1980; 746 p. (Gesammelte Werke 1. Abt.: Deutsche Schriften, Vol 8).

Wundt W. Grundzüge der physiologischen Psychologie. 4. Ausgabe, Vol. 1, Leipzig: W. Engelmann, 1893; 600 p.

Documenta Ophthalmologica 71: 113–122, 1989.

Chevalier Taylor – Ophthalmiater Royal (1703–1772)

PATRICK TREVOR-ROPER
Park Square West 3, London, N.W.1, UK

Abstract. John Taylor was surgeon-oculist to King George II, and claimed to be Ophthalmiater Royal to the Pope and to the Emperor, along with a multitude of royalties, including a mythical Princess of Georgia and the Viceroy of the Indies. He was the first and last ophthalmologist to travel from court to court of Europe with a cavalcade of outriders and supporters; and although he was caricatured as a mountebank, there was an element of genius about him, and his innovations, especially in squint surgery, demand that he should not be forgotten.

The mid-eighteenth century was the great turning point in ophthalmology, as in so many other fields, for thereafter the whole pattern of ocular therapy was transformed by the flowering of the scientific revolution, and by the coincident evolution of cataract surgery. But the old order was not to be overturned without one final flourish, epitomised in the flamboyant genius of John Taylor of Norwich.

The 'Chevalier' Taylor was born in Norwich, then the third city in England, on August 16, 1703 (he tells us that: 'between eleven and one he first became acquainted with the glories of the sun'). There his father was a well-known surgeon, and of five generations of John Taylors, four were doctors and his three successors oculists. He attended the practise at St Thomas Hospital in London, 'regularly and diligently' (as Cheselden confirmed), passing his examinations 'with all becoming exactness', and while scarcely of age was appointed chief surgeon at Norwich.

In those days surgery had changed little since the days of Babylon, with a staple fare of amputations of our disposable extremities (limbs, foreskins and hair), bloodletting, and an occasional turn at trepanning skulls; and the cutting for stones was about the only novelty that had been added to their menu. There were then no purely ophthalmic specialists, so, like his mentor Cheselden, he started on lithotomies before establishing his reputation as a coucher of cataracts.

Encountering opposition at Norwich, in 1727 he set out on his travels, first through England, Scotland, Ireland and Wales, returning to London in 1733. In 1734 he went to France and Holland, and back to London in 1735. Then, next year, he returned to Paris, and from 1737 to 1742 toured through

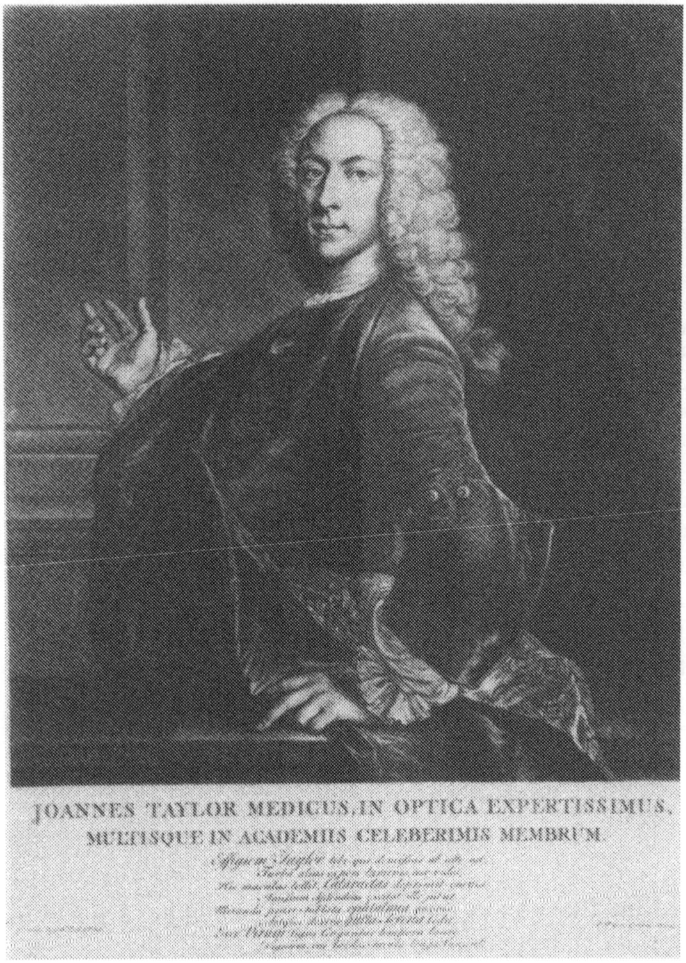
JOANNES TAYLOR MEDICUS, IN OPTICA EXPERTISSIMUS,
MULTISQUE IN ACADEMIIS CELEBERRIMIS MEMBRUM.

Fig. 1. John Taylor. J. Faber after Ryche. From the Wellcome Institute Library, London.

Spain and Portugal, where he is said to have celebrated his greatest triumphs. Then came another circuit of England, Scotland and Ireland before returning in 1747 to Holland and Flanders. In 1751 he was called to Rostock to restore the sight of the Duke of Mecklenburg-Schwerin, and visited Hamburg and Denmark, and during the following years he travelled 'day and night' through Sweden, Copenhagen, Breslau, Silesia, Warsaw, Mittau, Courland, Riga, St Petersburg and Moscow. He returned in 1755 through Germany and Bohemia to Italy, passing through Vienna and Ghent, and reaching London in 1758 or 1759. After another tour through Scotland, Ireland and Wales, he sedimented in London 'at Gravel Street,

Hatton Garden', where he published his *Travels and Adventures*, a fascinating, picaresque account; although the bones of this are clearly true there are many discrepancies between his own account of his itinerary and the facts, even when he had no apparent reason or intention to falsify. After this he announced his determination to enjoy a well-earned rest. But the wandering spirit was too strong for him. We catch a glimpse of him in 1765 at Amiens and Rheims, and one of his works was published in Hamburg and in Leipzig in 1766, and he reappeared in 1767 at Ghent. Of his last years we know little, except that he is said to have become blind before his death on June 6th, 1772 – in Paris (say some) or in a convent at Prague (according to his grandson). We know almost nothing of his private life, nor whether his wife and son accompanied him.

His epitaph (composed by himself, in what he calls 'his well-known peculiar manner', tells us that he had been eager only for the fame of others, had diligently sought the society of the learned, and found his highest joy in earning their friendship. In addition to some Latin verses (used elsewhere in his works), the following stanza is appended:

Dieux! Taylor git dans cette bière;
Cet oculiste si fameux;
Après avoir donné tant de fois la lumière,
Devait il donc fermer les Yeux!

During these journeys the Chevalier reckoned that he met everyone of note in the whole of Europe. Boerhaave 'continued me his correspondence and friendship to his latest hours', Haller had 'taken extraordinary pains to recommend me to the favour of the public', Morgagni was present when 'I was created doctor of Chirurgery in the University of Padua'; Winslow, Hunter, Monro and Linnaeus were numbered among his acquaintances. He travelled a hundred leagues to see Metastasio 'that no great man might escape me', and for the same reason, presumably, was on speaking terms with notorious criminals, including Mary Tofts, of Godalming, who persuaded even the King's surgeon, St André, that she had given birth to seventeen rabbits.

Honours and diplomas (he declared) were showered upon him. In 1734, after proving his abilities to the faculty, he was made a Fellow of the College of Physicians of Basel, and degrees were conferred upon him in Liège, Cologne and Rheims. Innumerable learned societies granted him testimonials or received him as a member. Municipalities presented him with sums of money. He held the office of 'ophthalmiater' to the Pope, the Emperor, and a multitude of Kings, Electors and Sovereign Princes, whose names were

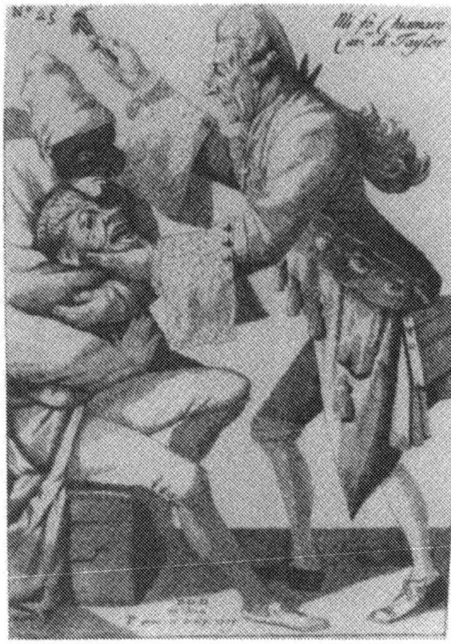

Fig. 2. John Taylor. Caricatured as a Mountebank in an etching by Thomas Patch, Florence.

listed in the title-page of some of his books, including the Duke of Mecklenburg, the Princess of Georgia, the Countess of Windischgraz, the illustrious Lady Nariskin, and Don A de Saldan, Viceroy of the Indies.

In all this extravagant boasting there is, undoubtedly, a kernel of truth. His objectionable methods were not the growth of a day, and there seems no reason to doubt that he did, in fact, receive degrees from several universities – the smaller ecclesiastical, rather than the larger, more scientific, schools (says Stricker). His claim to have been appointed oculist to George II in 1736 at least can be verified in our Public Records of 1736.

The Scots' Magazine for 1744 notes that: 'Dr Taylor, who has visited Glasgow and is returned, has caused register in the books of council and session, his diplomas as Doctor of Medicine by the Universities of Basel and Rheims in 1734, and by those of Liège and Cologne in 1735, also a certificate of his having been duly admitted oculist in ordinary to His Majesty in 1736'.

As to illustrious patients, his claim is well founded at least in the case of the Duke of Mecklenburg. He asserts that he operated on Bach and Händel, the former, 'at Leysick, where a celebrated master of music, who had already arrived at his 88th year, received his sight at my hands'; in Händel's case he hoped to have the like success, 'but, upon drawing the curtain, we found the bottom defective, from a paralytic disorder'. These statements contain ample inaccuracies: Bach never did attain his 88th year; he did not receive his sight but became blind after operation; Händel's operation had already been performed by Sharp in 1751, and again by Bromfield in 1752, and though the operation was unsuccessful he did not become completely blind. Taylor even asserts that Händel was educated by Bach, whereas, in fact, they never met. Gibbon also mentioned (in his autobiography) that he was treated by Taylor, but this is not included in Taylor's aristocratic list.

These public and professional triumphs, however, are colourless compared with some of the private adventures Taylor records. On one occasion a princess disguised herself as a poor girl and stopped him on the roadside, in order to discover if he were truly charitable, an ordeal from which the Chevalier declares that he emerged gloriously. At a masked ball he made love to a lady, who after two hours assured him of a 'reciprocal return'; and at the hour of unmasking she stood revealed as the Hereditary Princess of the Court.

In affairs of gallantry he was an acknowledged authority, and was often consulted by 'very great personages'. He tells us that he "once ventured abroad a little piece in Italian on 'The Art of making Love with Success'"; and also that 'the lady is not living on this side of forty, but on fixing my eyes upon her, I can read her very soul'. In fact, the wiser the lady the more likely was she to succumb, because she would be the better able to appreciate the Chevalier's wit. One one occasion he received an offer of marriage from a wealthy lady of 90, but discreetly misunderstood her meaning. His portraits confirm that he was a man of good personal appearance, and his grandson also testifies that he was a 'tall, handsome man, and a great favourite with the ladies'.

His more prosaic adventures were variegated. He had seen Jews burned, and knew all the secrets of the Inquisition; he had witnessed the various species of torture and methods of embalming, had studied the practice of inoculation in all lands, had met gipsies and hermits, and conformed to their manner of life. He was robbed on the frontiers of Spain and Portugal, and also between Naples and Rome, where he lost 'pictures of crowned heads, encircled with brilliants, instruments of solid gold, etc, to the value of 30,000 Roman crowns', and barely escaped with his life; but he received from the authorities a certificate of his misfortune, which served as an excellent advertisement.

The response of the medical profession to Taylor's flamboyant and boastful self-advertising was predictably harsh. Even in his early Norwich days he was censured, but his views on ophthalmology were considered with fairness by Duddell, one of his most distinguished seniors; and his reception by the continental eye surgeons was mixed. But it soon became common knowledge that his surgical results were generally disastrous. He tried to conceal these, for as soon as the operation was done, 'il chantoit victoire, il crioit un miracle' (Guérin), requiring the eye to be bandaged for five or six days, and after levying his spoils, decamped on the fourth. Dr Johnson declared that 'Taylor was the most ignorant man I ever knew, but sprightly', and that he was 'an instance of how far impudence can carry ignorance'.

Apart from these graver estimates, it is not surprising that he attracted a

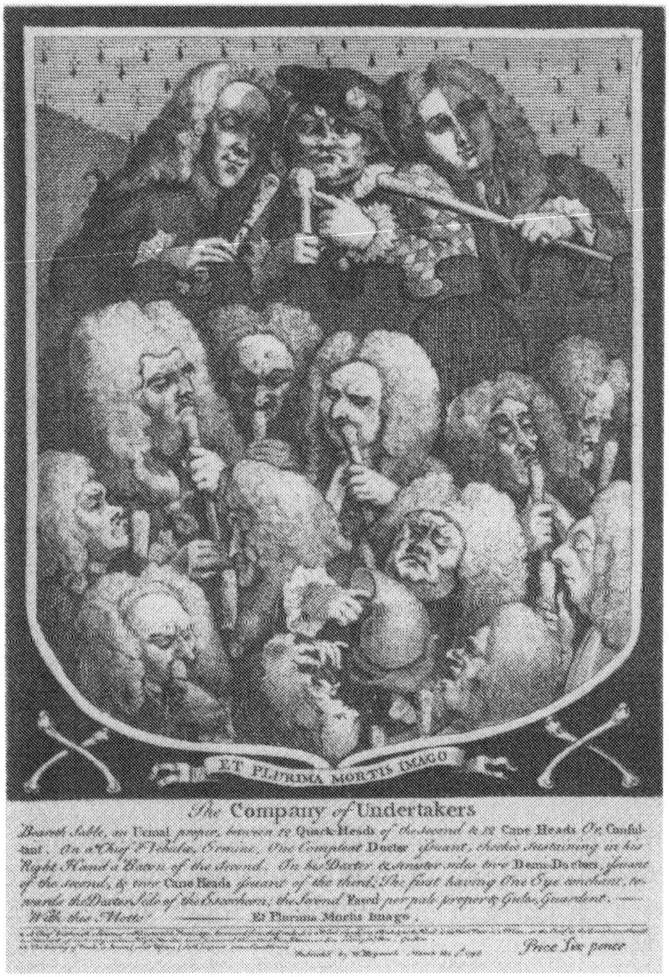

Fig. 3. 'The Company of Undertakers'. Cartoon by William Hogarth, 1736, featuring Taylor (top left) ogling his co-charlatan Mrs Mapp, as they peer from the gallery at the twelve physicians. From the Wellcome Institute Library, London.

shower of pasquinades, lampoons and squibs of all kinds, from London, Edinburgh and Dublin, including a 'ballad opera' in which Taylor figures as 'Dr Hurry, an oculist'. Again and again he is ridiculed in the company of Mrs Mapp (or Crazy Sally, the bonesetter) and Ward, the inventor of Ward's pill (Fig. 3); thus (from the Daily Journal of 16 November, 1736):

Three famous Quacks in one country born,
Epsom, Pallmall and Suffolk-street adorn:
M-p makes the Lame to walk by manuel slight;
T-r alike restores the Blind to Sight,
The Stone, the Gout, the P-x, and every ill
W-d cures internally by Drop and Pill.
Ye Quacks in Medicine prescribe no more;
Without it, these, as sure as Death, can cure.

After his death, his son planned a 'plain, unvarnished account of Taylor's life'. But being unversed in writing he passed the materials to Henry Jones, a disreputable Irish dramatist, who lost them during an unavoidable midnight change of lodgings. As the publication had already been announced, the 'profligate scribbler' concocted a ribald version from the odd bits he could remember and his own malicious invention.

During all these years of travel, Taylor published at least twenty treatises or monographs, with a similar number of reports and notices. These were published in Latin, English, French, German, Italian, Spanish, Portuguese, Danish, Swedish and Russian; in fact, books are still extant in the first five of these languages, and there seems no doubt that the main body of his works is his own, all of them having similar style, and the same views and opinions, even on minor matters.

The best remembered are the bombastic non-medical outpourings, especially those found in his dedicatory and prefatory letters and in his autobiography – 'History of the Travels and Adventures of the Chevalier John Taylor, Ophthalmiater', dedicated to his son and published in London in 1761. In this it is the mountebank who talks, using his most inflated style, with scant regard for truth, as shown in the following short extract:

Oh! ye imperial; oh! ye royal; oh! ye great masters of empire; who have so far extended your benevolence as to be witnesses of my labours . . . How often have you condescended to behold the transports that affected the mind, when from before the dark eye, by my hands, the dismal veil was removed, the curtain drawn; and saw, by my labours, this beauteous little globe re-assume its native power, and was again a lucid

> orb! Who then can suppose that you . . . would point out, as it were with the sceptre in hand, me alone amongst all mankind for these things, but from the strongest evidence that could be possibly desired for the support of truth?

In the rest of his works, especially the earlier ones, this posturing is absent, and he writes in plain English, with a sound knowledge of his subject and some originality in his observations and comments, even if his 'discoveries' are often borrowed from other authors. His early treatise 'An account of the Mechanism of the Eye' (Norwich 1727) is remarkably free from immoderate claims, and acknowledges that he is wholly indebted to Cheselden for his knowledge, and that his theory of vision derives from the writings of Bishop Berkeley a generation earlier.

Taylor's description of the Anatomy of the Eye simply and fairly reflects current knowledge, but his accounts of Ocular Physiology and Optics are of more interest. Hypermetropia and Myopia (attributed to altered convexity of the cornea) are clearly described, along with their correction by convex and concave glasses. The chiasmal crossing is understood, and the connection of the retinas with the nerve-centres is nicely likened to a bell-rope which has two ends (half of each optic nerve, so that a pull on either or both ends will ring the bell). He interprets accomodation correctly, reckoning that the lens 'perhaps assumes a different convexity' in order to see objects at different distances; but later, after a faulty observation that accomodation is retained after couching, he abandons his earlier view, believing that the lens was pulled forwards and backwards, not (as was then maintained) by muscle fibres in the ciliary ligament, but by pressure of the extraocular muscles, causing an elongation of the globe and increased corneal convexity.

He appreciates much of the significance of the pupil responses, including the consensual reaction (previously noted by Boerhaave), and the occasional association of mobile pupils with blindness – which he noted to be a sequel to dropsy or to loss of blood (from the brain's incapacity to receive impressions). He still believed that the choroid was the visual organ, but this is carefully discussed and in great detail, with the facts well marshalled (including arguments drawn from his interpretation of muscae volitantes as being evidences of retinal arterial distension).

Cataract was by then generally accepted to be an affection of the lens, with which Taylor fully concurred, although much argument continued over the nature of pupillary membranes. But he believed that cataract might be the sequel to a blow, violent greed, or the unskilful treatment of an ophthalmia (if the discharge, instead of being 'allured forwards by Kind Discutients' is 'drove back by cold Repellents'), and that the opacity reflected a viscidity of the blood, which prevented nourishing particles from passing through the lens pores. He later developed a theory that the cause was pressure of the external muscles from prolonged fixation on objects in a constant direction. He recognised the danger of operating on milky cataracts, and also on unilateral cataracts (because of the risk of losing both eyes); however, his cupidity overcame his judgement when he boasted of his 'new method of removing cataracts at all time, and in every species, without any Inflammation or the Possibility of an Accident'. The technique of couching he discusses in detail (opening the capsule below, and pressing the lens matter through the opening, as described by Petit), and he included ways of preserving the ciliary (ie suspensory) ligament, since it was perhaps responsible for accomodation. Because of the latter misconception, he rarely bothered with aphakic glasses; and in any event, he rarely tarried long enough to witness the consequences of his surgery. It was suggested that Taylor actually performed cataract extraction before Daviel, but he probably just followed the current practise of removing, through a corneal incision, lenses which had become dislocated into the anterior chamber on attempted couching or when the uncouchable soft cataracts had become broken up; and indeed he was roundly critical of Daviel's method, only admitting to performing this operation many years later (in 1765).

For Amaurosis or Gutta Serena, he was unable to resist offering treatment – pricking the eye-muscles or rubbing the eyeball so as to persuade the fixed pupil to move (since 'it is on the natural movements of the pupil that depends the healthful Protection of Sight').

Concerning Squint, Taylor's views were indeed in advance of his time, classifying the different presentations, appreciating that squint could derive from poor acuity and that the image was simply suppressed in the squinting eye; he also understood that some squints were sequels to lesions of the eye muscles. He certainly considered tenotomy of the superior oblique, the internal rectus or division of their nerve supply, but was rather secretive about the actual technique he used.

Iritis he accepted as a precursor of occluded pupil; and he knew the risk of sympathetic uveitis (he warned against surgery in unilateral cataract, lest both eyes be lost). Corneal opacities were sometimes pared off if protuberant or scrubbed with a small brush. Ptosis and ectropion also yielded to his suturing (in both of his patients, being young ladies of fashion, his accounts are very suspect). Conical cornea was correctly identified. Glaucoma was then a barely conceived disease of the lens, which Taylor thought was actually due to a swelling of it.

So the 'Chevalier' Taylor remains as a picturesque milestone in ophthalmic history, of good address and appearance, confident and engaging. He was an unparalleled liar and pre-eminent charlatan; his naturally grand manner, reflected in his flamboyant advertising, was helped by a quiet wit and ready turn of phrase. But his knowledge was impressive, and he was a shrewd observer, equipped with originality, energy and industry. All of this lifted him far above the retinue of rogues and charlatans which have plagued medicine since prehistory.

Notes

My account relies heavily on the biographical details provided by George Coats, published in the Royal London Ophthalmic Hospital Reports (Vol. 20) of May 1915, in which Taylor's complete bibliography is listed along with copious references. A concise biographical account, with that of his son, is also found in the Dictionary of National Biography (Vol. 55) 1898.

Documenta Ophthalmologica 71: 123–141, 1989.

Santiago Ramón Y Cajal, the retina and the neuron theory

MARCO PICCOLINO, ENRICA STRETTOI & ELENA LAURENZI
Istituto di Fisiologia Generale dell'Universita' di Ferrara Italy, and Istituto di Neurofisiologia del C.N.R. di Pisa, Italy

Received October 1988

> 'A small block of nervous tissue left from several days, hardening in Müller fluid alone or mixed with osmic acid. Because the histologist was distracted, or because of a scientist's curiosity, it was immersed in a bath of silver nitrate. One sections the block, dehydrates the sections, clears them, and examines them. Surprising sight! Against a perfectly translucent, yellow background, appear, thinly dispersed, the black filaments, either smooth and delicate or spiny and thick; the black cell bodies, triangular, stellate, fusiform. They might be drawings done with India ink on transparent Japanese vellum. One is taken aback; the eye is accustomed to the inextricable tangles seen in sections stained with carmine or hematoxylin, where the mind strains in prodigies of criticism and interpretation, always in doubt. Here everything is simple, clear without confusion. Nothing more to interpret. One only needs to see and to record this cell with multiple ramified branches, covered with a fuzz like hoarfrost and encompassing with their undulations an astonishingly large space; or this smooth and uniform fiber, which arises from the cell, extending for enormous distances, and suddenly bursting into a spray of budding fibers; or that cell body confined to the ventricular wall and sending a process to ramify at the very surface of the brain; or other stellate cells, resembling feather starfish or the daddy-longlegs; amazed, the eye cannot break off from looking! The dream technique is a reality! The metallic impregnation has produced a subtle dissection, more than one dared hope for. This is the Golgi method' [1].

With these words in 1909 [2], Santiago Ramón y Cajal (Fig. 1, 2) described with a sense of drama and high emotion, the enchantment aroused by preparations of the nervous tissue obtained with the chromo-argentic technique, the famous "*reazione nera*" discovered by Camillo Golgi in 1873 [2]. In his autobiography, Cajal mentions even the address of the laboratory in Madrid where in 1887, for the first time, he saw histological sections prepared according to the method of the celebrated scientist of Pavia (at the '*Calle del Arco de Santa Maria*', number 41). At that time, Cajal was a young professor of anatomy at the university of Valencia (he was born in 1852). He could have spent his life 'vegetating sadly in a provincial university without passing in the scientific order beyond the category of more or less estimable delvers after details' [3]. But suddenly the year 1888 arrived, 'the year of fortune' which was a milestone in an extraordinary scientific adventure whose fruits were to lay firm foundations for neuroanatomy and, more generally, for all studies of the nervous system. Against all expectations, a long-cherished dream was realized, 'the rather chimerical idea of building up histology in Spain in spite of the indifference, when there was not hostility, of the intellectual atmosphere' [3].

One century ago, in 1888, Cajal published the first results of his studies

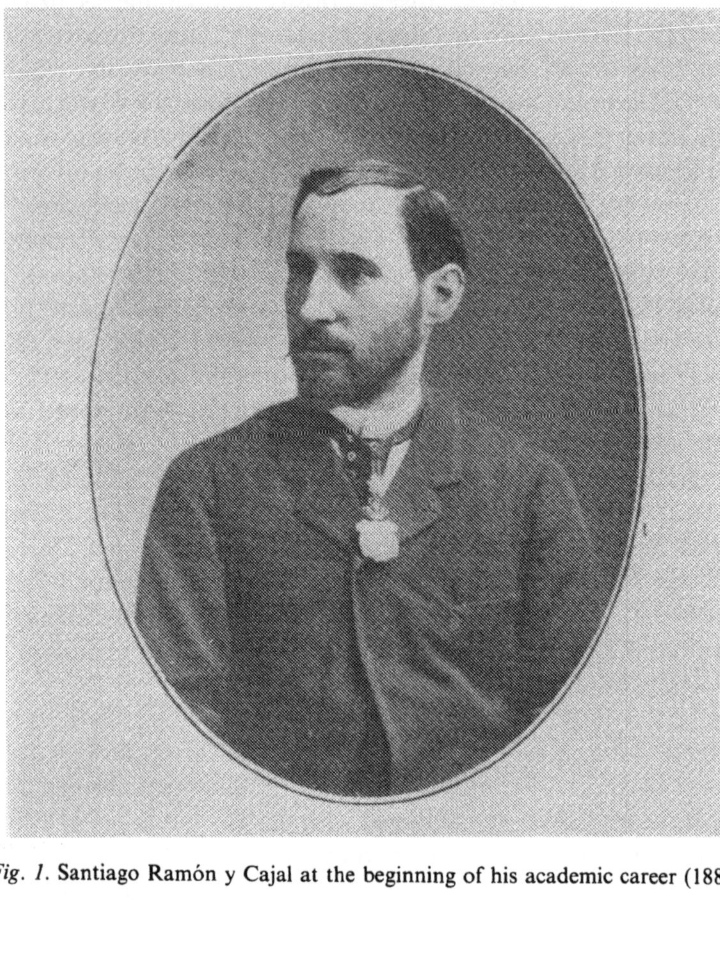

Fig. 1. Santiago Ramón y Cajal at the beginning of his academic career (1884).

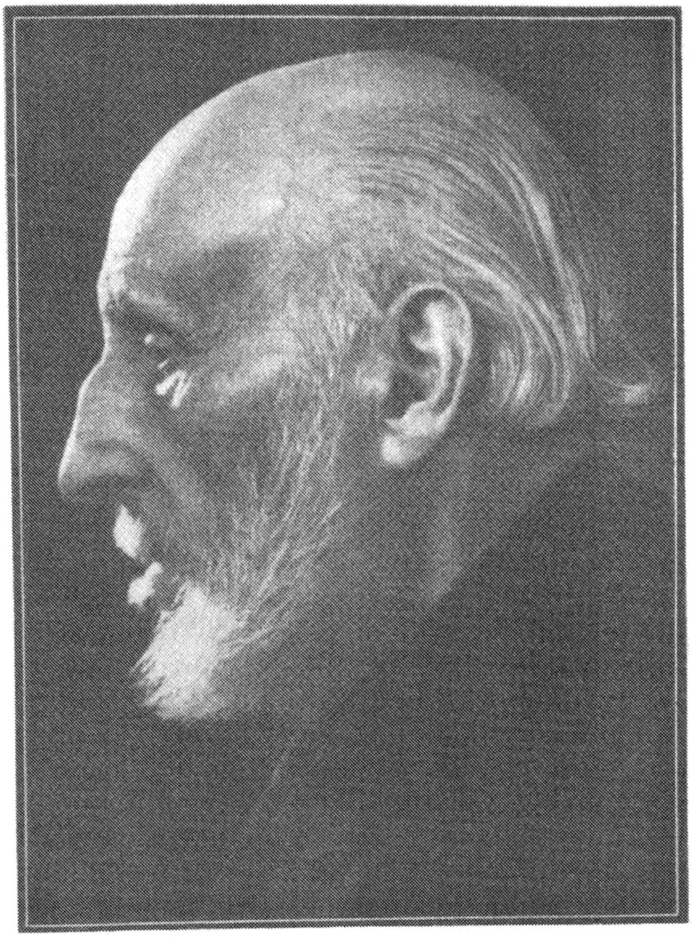

Fig. 2. Santiago Ramón y Cajal in one of the last photos of his life (From Cajal, 1923).

carried out with the Golgi method, studies which he had undertaken in a 'feverish ardour' on his return to Valencia after the short visit to Madrid where he had become acquainted with the new technique [4–7]. With an illuminating intuition, Cajal assumed that the elegant structures appearing most clearly in the Golgi preparations were nothing but the nerve cells, stained in their entirety, 'coloured brownish black even to their finest branchlets' [3]. Interpreting on this base the results of his studies, Cajal soon realized that they contradicted in some fundamental points the prevailing theories on the structural organization of the nervous system. In the cerebellum he observed that the axons of nerve cells came in contact with the dendrites and cell bodies of other nerve cells, but he saw that each cell retained in the contact its individuality ('the fortunate discovery of the *terminal baskets* and of climbing fibers' [3], Fig. 3); the "reticular theory" of Gerlach [8] viewed the arborizations of nerve cells establishing anastomoses with each another in a relation of true continuity, giving rise to a single overlying network permeating the whole nervous system. Golgi, somewhat modifying the initial conception of Gerlach, assumed that the dendritic arborizations did not enter in the constitution of this network, (his "rete nervosa diffusa"). He had shown that the dendrites end in the gray matter with free endings, and he supposed that dendrites and cell bodies were not involved in nervous conduction, but instead had a pure trophic function [9]. In contrast to the views of Gerlach and Golgi, Cajal's observations on the cerebellum showed the absence of any protoplasmic continuity between nervous elements; moreover, the existence of contacts between the axonal terminals on the one side, and the cell bodies or dendrites on the other, implied a conductive role also for dendrites and cell bodies, and contradicted Golgi's hypothesis of their exclusively trophic function.

The reasons why Golgi and other scientists adhered to the reticular theory may be found in part in the great influence exerted in the 19th century by the "non-localist" conception of the nervous function [10] supported by the studies and the authority of the French physiologist Pierre Flourens. In opposition to the "phrenology" of Franz Gall and Johan Spurzheim, who favoured an extreme localization of the cerebral functions, Flourens supported the fundamental unity of the brain.

In the opinion of Flourens, 'from the physiological point of view the brain is a unit carrying out the same functions in its totality as well in its components' [11].

Golgi quoted this sentence in an article published in 1891 in which he discussed his theory of the "Rete nervosa diffusa" [12]. In the same article, he mentioned the famous experiments of Friedrich Goltz, the physiologist of Strasbourg, who in those same years showed how important motor functions persisted in the dog after extensive cerebral ablations [13].

For Golgi, the brain activity involved the existence of an "... intimate relation between the function of the different parts of the nervous system; intimate relation having the character of reciprocity". And his "rete nervosa diffusa" appears to be suited to 'connect functionally the different parts' of the nervous system, and, at the same time, it 'seems in such contrast with the conception of the precise cerebral localizations that we would be brought to reject completely the doctrine of localizations' [12].

Contrary to the expectations of the reticular theory, the results of Cajal's

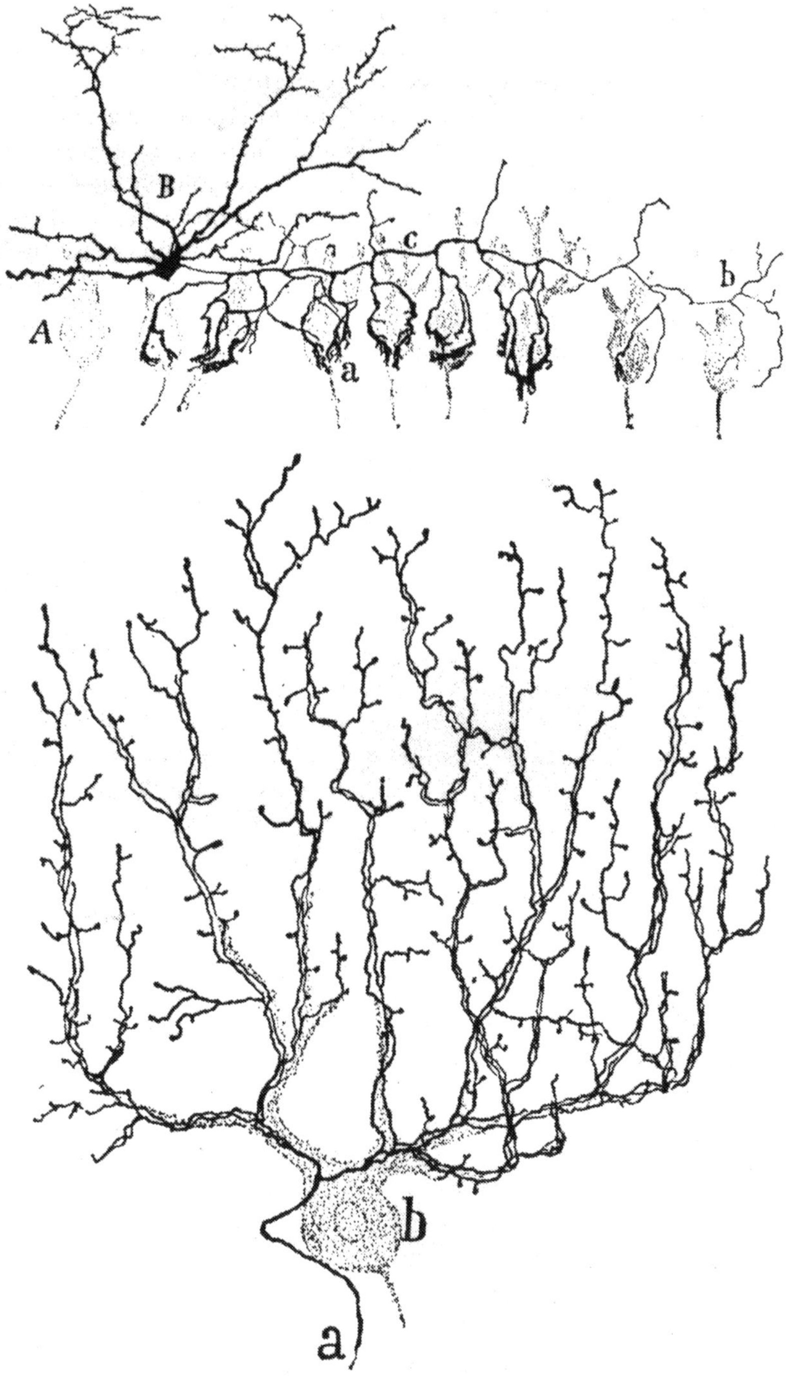

Fig. 3. Basket cell (A) and climbing fiber (B), impregnated with the Golgi method, and their connections with Purkinje cells. (From Cajal, ref. 1).

first studies in the cerebellum pointed toward a "cellular" conception of the nervous system. As a matter of fact, a cellular hypothesis had been proposed in those same years by A.H. His and W. Forel [14–15], who suggested that the transmission between nerve cells could occur in the absence of protoplasmic anastomoses. The hypothesis of His and Forel suited well the experimental observations of Cajal, but did not satisfy completely his demand for an understanding of the general plan of organization of nervous centers.

In contrast to Golgi, Cajal believed that the nervous functions '(reflexes, instinctive actions, functional localizations in the brain) demand imperiously the recognition of perfectly circumscribed paths or channels of conduction through the cerebrospinal axis'.

From Cajal's standpoint, the fatal consequence of any theory which affirms a diffuse bidirectional communication between nerve elements, by contact or continuity, is that it leads ineluctably to an 'indeterminacy of the path of nervous vibration ..., to declaring the absolute unsearchability of the organ of the soul' [3], the brain.

Cajal had an instinctive aversion to the idea that in the nervous system 'everything communicates with everything' in a sort of 'protoplasmic

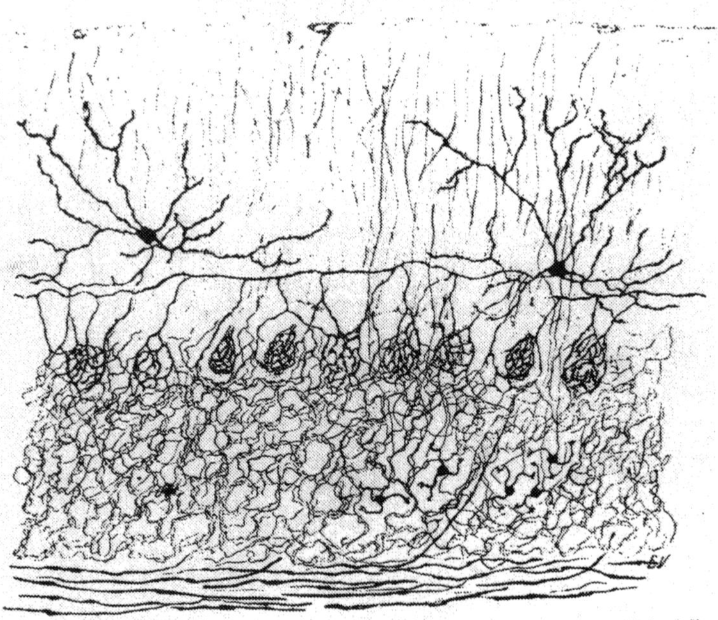

Fig. 4. Cerebellar cortex which shows the connections between the basket cells and the Purkinje cells, and illustrates the constitution of "rete nervosa diffusa". Golgi method. (From Golgi, published in Luciani, ref. 44).

pantheism' [3]. In the cerebellum, Cajal had divined a plan of orderly connectivity, by noting the absence of certain types of contact (reciprocal contacts between dendrites, or between axons), and by revealing exclusively axo-somatic and axo-dendritic contacts (see Fig. 3). In his mind the idea began to emerge that a correct interpretation of this connectivity scheme might prove to be decisive.

Cajal next studied the retina, wishing to confirm, by an elucidation of its organization, the general validity of his observations, and looking for a principle capable of disentangling the complexity of cerebral circuits. Cajal considered the visual membrane, the retina, as 'a true nervous center, as a peripheral extension of the central nervous system ... especially suitable for histological analysis'. In his opinion 'a study of the retina would shed light on the general problem of the connection and mechanism of action of nervous cells' [16].

'If an organ exists about which we know in a satisfactory way the paths of nervous impulses, this is the visual membrane. The simplest analysis of the arrangement of retinal articulations shows us that the nervous wave propagates in the retina from behind to forward, perpendicularly to its layers, the impulse arising in cones and rods, and passing afterward to the bipolar and ganglionic elements' [17].

In his studies on the avian retina published in 1888 [6,7], Cajal showed that in this structure the cells connect with each other by contact, without protoplasmic anastomoses. Moreover, as in the cerebellum, the contacts are found exclusively between axon endings on one side, and dendritic arborizations and cell bodies on the other.

The studies on the retina continued in the following years, and provided results which were fundamental for Cajal's formulation of his principles of the general organization of nervous connections [16,17–19]. Beside affirming that the nervous tissue is made up on independent elements, the neurons (so named in 1891 by Wilhelm Waldeyer [20]), Cajal proposed the principle of dynamic polarization:

'The transmission of nervous movement takes place from the protoplasmic branches, (the dendrites), and from the cell body to the nervous expansion, (the axon). In this respect, every nerve cell possesses a receptor apparatus (the cell body and the protoplasmic expansions), an apparatus of conduction (the cylinder-axis), and an apparatus of emission (the terminal varicose arborization of the cylinder-axis)' [21].

In order to understand the interpretative value of this principle, we must take into account that in Cajal's time there were few electrophysiological studies on the pathways followed by the nervous signal within the cerebral circuits. With Cajal's principle at hand, in order to trace the pathway of signal transmission along the central circuits, it sufficed to identify the somato-dendritic region and the axon of the constituent neurons and the arrangement of their contacts.

His interest in the retina never abandoned Cajal, as he recognized in his memoirs '... the retina has always shown to be generous with me ... the retina the oldest and most tenacious of my laboratory loves ...' [3].

The scheme of general organization of the retina proposed by Cajal is still valid in its fundamental outline, and in several aspects Cajal studies remain 'the most outstanding and comprehensive descriptions of retinal structure' [22]. The retina, previously regarded as an inextricable membrane consisting of reticular and granular layers of uncertain significance, with Cajal became a true nervous structure where specific classes of nerve cells connect with other nerve cells, in order to convey the visual message toward the encephalic centers, along well defined pathways (Fig. 5).

The specific contributions of Cajal to the study of the retina are numerous. Among others there were the description of several morphological types of bipolar, amacrine and ganglion cells, the identification of different sublaminae in the inner plexiform layer, the discovery of the centrifugal fibers in the optic nerve, the identification of the circuit of efferent control in the retina, the description of the interplexiform cells (his small stellate cells of teleosts and mammals), in addition to the detailed description of Müller cells (see in particular ref. 16 and 19); moreover, Cajal's contributions to retinal histogenesis were of fundamental importance.

Although the work on the retina was so fruitful and important in the scientific life of Cajal, we should not think that it developed along a pathway devoid of obstacles. In fact, the difficulties and the polemics that Cajal encountered were many. Moreover, in some cases his observations and conclusions do not appear to be well supported by solid experimental evidence.

The difficulties and uncertainties of Cajal do not cast a shadow on the work of the great Spanish scientist. In our opinion they constitute an element of great interest because their analysis offers an insight not only into Cajal's personality, but also into the psychology of the investigative process in science.

Clear difficulties in Cajal's work on the retina concern the general plan of the connection between nerve cells. In Cajal's view, the retina is organized according to a scheme of point-to-point transmission of the visual message. That message, which originates in photoreceptors, should be conveyed by the most direct anatomical pathway to the brain so as to create a faithful neural copy of the optical image. Any excessive convergence in nervous pathways, and any lateral propagation of retinal circuits, appear to be potentially dangerous, since they could lead to a weakening or to a loss of the power of spatial discrimination. In many of his diagrams on the flow of visual messages in the retina, Cajal only showed the chain formed by photoreceptors – bipolar cells – ganglion cells, thus excluding systematically other retinal neurons (Fig. 5).

In the retina there are at least two classes of neurons which, by their anatomical arrangement in a tangential plane, seem to be organized expressly for a lateral flow of information: the horizontal and the amacrine cells; moreover, the wide dendritic arborisations of some classes of bipolar and ganglion cells are suggestive of great functional convergence.

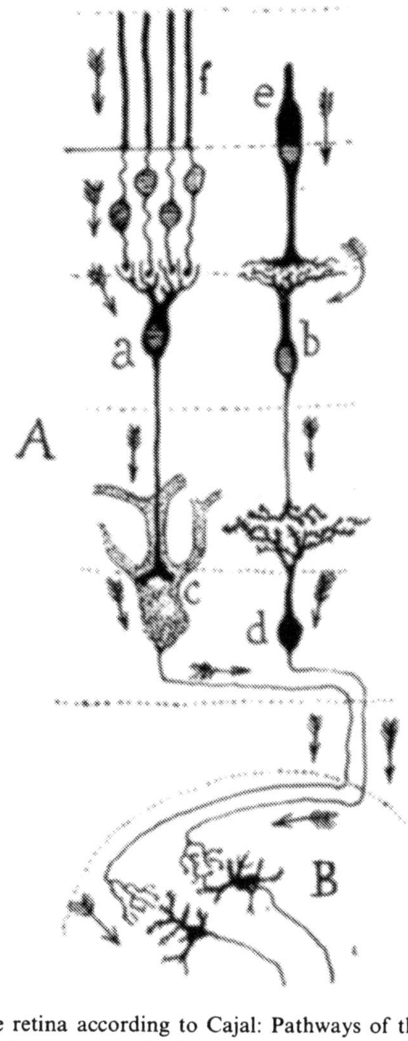

Fig. 5A. Scheme of the retina according to Cajal: Pathways of the nervous impulse in the vertebrate retina up to the geniculate body.

Insofar as amacrine cells are concerned, Cajal seems to exclude that these neurons receive the visual input from the bipolar cells, and he assumes that they are involved uniquely in a circuit of efferent control (centrifugal fibers of optic nerve – amacrine cells – ganglion cells, Fig. 5b). In this way, Cajal can account also for the wide dendritic arborisations of some ganglion cells, by supposing that these structures serve to receive the signal conveyed by amacrine cells along the efferent circuit. The large ganglion cells would receive the "visual" message mainly in the region of the soma, from a small number of bipolar cells (Fig. 5c and b). Such an arrangement has not been confirmed by modern studies, which, on the contrary, underline the scarcity, or even the absence, of any synaptic input from bipolar cells onto the ganglion cell body. Furthermore, in mammals, the bipolars that Cajal assumes to end on the ganglion cell body (rod bipolars) actually do not make any contact with ganglion cells, and send their visual message to these cells exclusively through a subset of amacrine cells. A second possibility considered by Cajal in order to account for the existence of extensive convergence on the large ganglion cells, while preserving the analytical

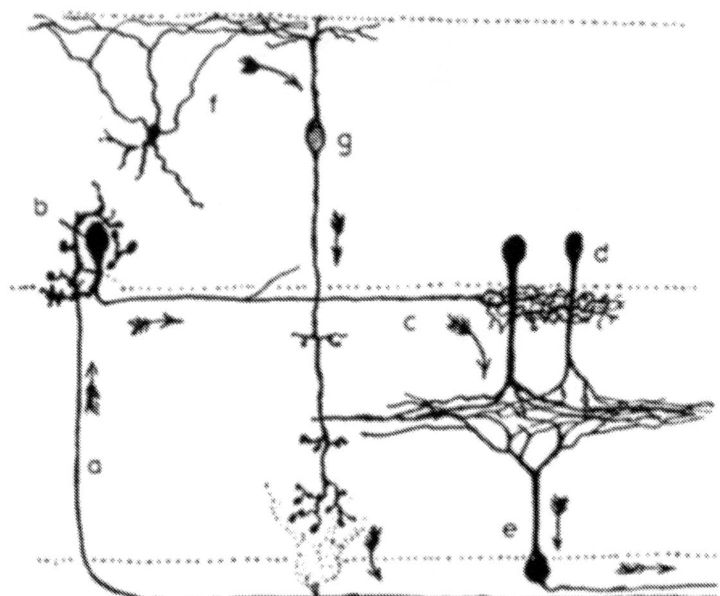

Fig. 5B. Scheme of the retina according to Cajal. Efferent circuit in the avian retina: (a, efferent, retinopetal, fiber of optic nerve: b e c, the so-called association amacrine with its axon; d, ordinary amacrine; e, ganglion cell; f, small stellate cell (now denoted as interplexiform); g, bipolar cell.

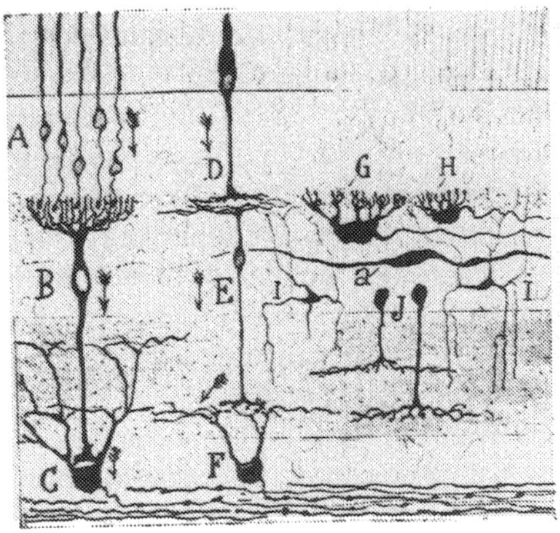

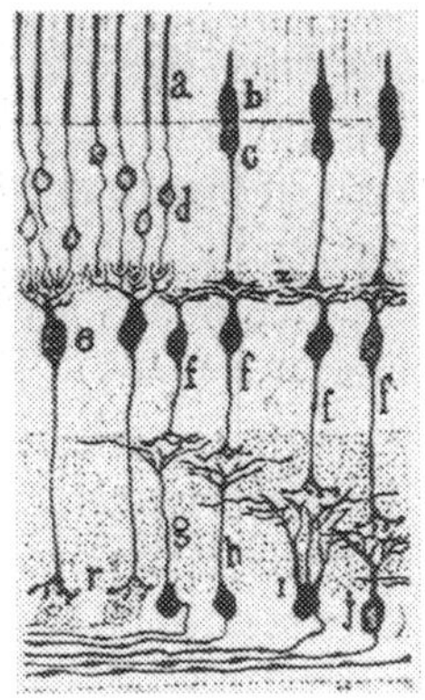

Fig. 5C. Fish retina: A, rods; B e C, bipolar and ganglion cells for rods; D, cone; E e F, bipolar and ganglion cell for cones; G, H, horizontal cells; I, small stellate cells (interplexiform); J, amacrine cell; a, horizontal cell axon-terminal which Cajal thought to be a subtype horizontal cells.

Fig. 5D. Channel of transmission of the signal from rods (a) and from cones (b) in the mammal retina (from Cajal, ref. 3).

power of visual perception, was to assume that these cells were involved exclusively in the pathways of visual reflexes (as opposed to the pathway of the 'mental visual image' [1]) where convergence should be minimal.

The problem of convergence concerns also the bipolar cells. And for these cells, the possibility existed, as suggested by other histologists, that the signal from both cones and rods would converge on the same bipolar cell. Cajal, who adhered to the duplicity theory of Max Schultze, according to which cones and rods mediate respectively the diurnal, chromatic, vision and the nocturnal, achromatic, vision, refused this convergence because:

'. . . the ingenious expedient according to which nature has organized two classes of specific photoreceptor cells would be completely frustrated: since, from the second neuron onward, both impressions, that of colour and that of black and white, would have to combine as they ran together through the same channels' [3].

And thus he began to explore eagerly the retina looking for bipolar cells specific for the transmission of the two types of signals, profoundly convinced that:

'When we reason with common sense and lift the war club determined upon vigorous action, nature ultimately hears us' [3]; and in fish and mammals eventually he found what he was looking for, bipolar for cones distinct from bipolar for rods:

'... and finally, as the reward of my faith, there deigned to appear most clearly and brilliantly those two types of bipolar cells demanded by theory and divined by reason' [3] (Fig. 5c and d).

It is clear from these words that in Cajal the "object" of the research may somewhat "precede" the experimental observations, and it can be guessed on the basis of theoretical conceptions or general principles. As a matter of fact, recent studies, while confirming the existence of separate rod and cone bipolars in mammals, lead us to reconsider the idea of a clear distinction between the two types of bipolars in fish. Moreover, it appears that even in mammals there is a clear convergence at the ganglion cell level of signals coming from the classes of photoreceptors [23–24].

Many difficulties and problems arose for Cajal in the interpretation of the cellular organization and functional significance of horizontal cells.

Surprisingly, Cajal ignored in a systematic way the presence, in the retinas of most species, of an axonless type of horizontal cell [16], in spite of the fact that the existence of such neurons had been reported by other authors. And this even when histological research could take advantage of neurofibrillar methods, which, in the retina of many mammals, mainly stain axonless cells [17]. One is led to conceive that Cajal saw exclusively axon-bearing horizontal cells because these conformed well to the principle of dynamic polarization.

As for horizontal cells (and other retinal neurons), another series of problems concerned the possible existence of intercellular, protoplasmic anastomoses. These had been reported by other authors (Krause, Dogiel), but Cajal refuted them with vigour [1,16–17,19]. In particular Tartuferi, the first to apply the Golgi method to the retina [25], claimed the existence of extensive anastomoses between horizontal cells, as well as between photoreceptor endings, thus creating an overspread network ("rete sottoepiteliale"), beneath photoreceptors. Anastomoses were also reported by other histologists using neurofibrillar methods [26]. Although in this case Cajal guessed correctly the discrete character of horizontal cells, we must take into account that the histological appearance was not unequivocal in that respect. As a matter of fact, only electron microscopy could give a definite answer to this problem, due to the narrow space existing between neighbouring neurons.

Moreover, in the case of horizontal cells, recent studies have pointed the syncytial character of their organization. Adjacent cells may be interconnected by wide and numerous gap junctions. These junctions consist of hydrophilic channels which allow for the transcellular passage of ions and small molecules between connected cells [27–28]. In the case of some horizontal cell types, because of these junctions, the functional unit does not correspond to the individual cells, as visualized by Golgi preparations; it corresponds better to the intricate syncytium stained with neurofibrillar methods, or to the images obtained following intracellular injection in one cell of low molecular-weight dyes that spread between cells to illuminate a network of connected neurons [29–30]. This syncytium is somewhat reminiscent of the nerve network of the theories of Gerlach and Golgi.

In this context it is worth to point out here that gap junctions exist also between photoreceptors as well as between other retinal neurons [23–24,31]. Moreover, to emphasize the ambiguous appearance of the optical microscopy images, let us consider that the process of second order neurons may penetrate within the base of photoreceptors in the so-called invaginated synapses [32]. One could perhaps say that Tartuferi, in describing his "rete sottoepiteliale", recorded in a more faithful way the images of Golgi preparations. On the other hand, Cajal interpreted these images more correctly, since, supported by more adequate theoretical principles, he was able to see beyond the pure objective datum.

Coming back to horizontal cells, it is worth mentioning here that in the retinas of lower vertebrates the syncytial aspect of the terminal expansions of the axon-bearing horizontal cells is particularly remarkable. In the fish retina, such expansions are spindle-shaped and they form a continuous plexus layer lying internal to the horizontal cell bodies [33]. In preparations stained with the Golgi method it is extremely difficult to trace the entire course of the axon. Cajal was disconcerted by these anucleate structures. He described then the presence of nuclei in the axonal expansions, and considered them as a specific subset of horizontal cells ("internal horizontal cells", ref. 16, Fig. 5d). He even wondered why other authors were not able to see the presence of nuclei in these structures. For example, Schiefferdecker denoted them as "anucleate concentric cells ('kernlose concentrische Zellen') [34]. It is difficult to escape the conclusion that Cajal, in "seeing" the nucleus in the axonal expansions of fish horizontal cells may have corrected in a "cellular" sense an image that appeared to be in contrast with the postulates of neuronal theory.

With respect to the comprehension of the role of horizontal cells, many problems arose for Cajal, which were somewhat analogous to those regarding the amacrine cells. On the basis of his experimental observations, Cajal was brought to conclude that horizontal cells did not participate in the pathway of the "vertical" transmission of the visual message, and that they might establish connections between photoreceptors separated by long distances [1,16]. But then:

"we are obliged to admit that the visual signal seized by these tangential neurons flows back, toward the visual corpuscles of other visual radiations (the photoreceptors of other retinal regions), somewhat far away, such as to constitute a kind of vicious circle' [35].

A similar possibility was contrary to the conception of a plan of orderly and economic connectivity that Cajal supposed the structural scheme of organization of the nervous system in general, and of the retina in particular.

'May one admit that this would be a real association, in a transverse plane, of visual corpuscles. For a sensitive apparatus endowed with such an analytical power, is it ever possible to admit that nature has established an arrangement which implies the destruction of the differentiation power of cones and rods and which is capable of weakening or even suppressing in certain regions their spatial sign [1]?'

To solve what would remain for his entire life the 'paradox of horizontal cells' [35], Cajal assumes that the function of these cells was not to transmit the visual message from one point to another of the retina, but instead, that horizontal cells would serve as 'depot of nervous energy aimed at reinforcing visual excitation and giving it a tension sufficient to bring it up to the centers [1].' He applied to horizontal cells an a priori view that he had formulated to explain the presence and the functional role of neurons with short axons in many regions of the nervous system [36]. The study of horizontal cells had been rather decisive in the elaboration of this conception. Due to their anatomical characteristics, the short-axon neurons appeared to Cajal unsuited to "project" the electrical signal from one region to another. They seemed to be in many cases a redundant, or even functionally dangerous, element in the structural plan of the nervous tissue. For example, in the cerebellum, to assume that short-axon neurons are all involved in conduction pathways would lead to a variety of parallel or recurrent pathways that Cajal considered a 'superfluous complication' [36]. And in the retina, 'if horizontal cells were constantly interspersed between the two factors of nervous articulation (photoreceptors and bipolar cells), the physiological effect would be to disturb, or to hinder, the spatial function of every retinal point' [36].

On the other hand, Cajal believed that short-axon neurons played an important role since they are particularly abundant in nervous structures subserving higher functions (such as the cerebral and cerebellar cortices, the striatum), and their number increases along the phylogenetic axis, going from lower vertebrates to mammals and humans. And then he supposed that they would act as 'condensers or accumulators of nervous energy', whose discharge 'would contribute to increase the tension of the impulses flowing along the chain of the corpuscles with long axons' [1]. And, in a following passage, he concludes:

'In every action which takes place a long time after an excitation of internal origin (memory, ideation, judgement, etc.), the aforementioned cells would go on, giving up their dynamic reserve until, exhausted, tiredness would eventually arrive' [1].

The difficulties of Cajal in interpreting the physiological significance of short-axon neurons, and of some aspects of retinal organization, to a great extent were due to the absence, in his general principles, of an integrative and operational conception of nervous function. In the plan of orderly connectivity formulated by Cajal, it seems that the only function of nervous cells is to transmit visual signals from a site to another along well defined pathways, with a minimal number of neurons. It is interesting to note in this context that, according to Cajal, only two neurons (one sensory and the other motor) are sufficient to account for most of the spinal reflexes [1].

In particular, Cajal lacked the notion of inhibitory interaction between nerve cells as a fundamental operative mechanism in the central circuits. He was surprised by the phenomenon of inhibition in spinal reflexes which may occur in several functional circumstances (e.g., intense emotions, electrical stimulations of the contralateral side):

'As a matter of fact it appears rather strange that a powerful excitation results in a motor inhibition instead of eliciting extensive, coordinated reflexes and conscious reactions' [1].

And he assumed that this phenomenon was not a consequence of a true, active inhibition exerted by specific nervous pathways, but depended instead on an intrinsic incapacity of the spinal neuron to respond to excessive stimuli:

'In our opinion, the motor neuron is tuned to respond to a limited scale of stimulus intensities; if this scale is exceeded it shows itself unexcitable both for stimulation coming from the pyramidal tract, and for impulses arriving from sensitive and sensorial nerves' [1].

This absence of the notions of integration and inhibition in the interpretative paradigms of Cajal explains, for instance, his difficulty in accepting the presence of complex local circuits in the cerebellum.

This is also the reason why Cajal could not accept the possibility of a lateral flow of the retinal signal, a flow that, as we have already seen, he considered deleterious for the analytical requirements of the visual process.

The existence of lateral inhibition in the retina was first recognized by Hartline in *Limulus* in the late 1940s, and confirmed some year later by Barlow and Kuffler in vertebrates (see ref. 37). The studies that followed demonstrated that, through processes of lateral interaction, the retina carries out a complex analysis of the visual message. It does not simply generate and transmit a photographic replica of the optical stimulus [23,28,30].

If Cajal had supposed that horizontal cells, by connecting distant photoreceptors through recurrent, inhibitory pathways, could serve, not to deteriorate, but instead to *increase* the analytical power of visual process, certainly he would have had fewer problems in interpreting the structural plan of the retina (and of other nervous centers).

On the other hand, we must take into account that a great merit of Cajal was to recognize, within the apparent complexity of the nervous system, a basic structure accessible to anatomical and functional stuedy; this structure consists of nerve cells, which establish specialized contacts whereby nervous messages proceed along well-defined and circumscribed pathways. And Cajal did this in a period dominated by "anti-localicistic" and "holistic" conceptions of the nervous function. As a matter of fact, in spite of Cajal's statement that in Golgi preparations there was no more need for interpretation, but only to see and to take note of an unambiguous reality, the interpretation is always a fundamental phase in the acquisition of knowledge in science. The same experimental data can lead to conclusions which are diametrically opposed in the hands of two scientists, both endowed with an exceptional talent (Fig. 3A and Fig. 4). Where Cajal sees the axon of basket cells terminating with free endings that embrace the body of Purkinje cells, Golgi sees the axon terminals continuing in a "rete nervosa diffusa".

Integration and inhibition are physiological concepts which could not have emerged primarily from morphological studies. Their formulation in a modern sense is based on the notion of the synapse, which could develop only within the framework of a cellular theory of the nervous function. At the beginning of this century, the notion of the synapse entered the realm of neurobiology mainly due to the work of Sherrington, the great English physiologist, a devoted admirer of Cajal, who recognized the debt on the part of physiologists, to the studies of the great Spanish anatomist [39–40].

At the beginning of 20th century the neuron theory, and with it neurobiology at its inception, was faced by a violent attack delivered by new "reticularists". In particular the zoologist S. Apathy, and the physiologist A. Bethe, supported the notion that the neurofibrils, revealed in nervous cells by recently discovered methods, were the basic structure of the functional organization of the nervous system. By anastomosing with each another, and independently from nerve cells, which were relegated to secondary functions, the neurofibrils would serve to conduct the nervous signal, acting as tiny electrical wires [41–42].

Cajal was obliged to take sides in this polemic against a theory which was really dangerous, and he intervened with a vigour which was criticized. The polemics persisted until Cajal's death, at which time his final defense against old and new antineuronists was in press [43].

Without Cajal's propensity to simplify and to catch the essential in the observation and interpretation of histological images, no doubt the progress of neurobiology would have been delayed. We are now able to understand some minor limitations in his theories and conclusions without losing our faith in his fundamental achievements: we can now accept the idea that, in some cases, neurons form syncytia due to the presence of intercellular bridges; that the nervous signal can circulate along pathways in contrast with the doctrine of dynamic polarization, and that there exist dendro-dendritic or axo-axonic synapses; that in nervous centers there are complex local circuits. We can now accept, and try to understand, the complex and variable nature of neuronal circuits having learned from Cajal what is simple and constant therein.

Acknowledgements

The authors wish to thank Paul Witkovsky for critically reading the manuscript and helping with the English translation.

References and notes

1. Ramón y Cajal S (1909–1911) Histologie du Système Nerveux de l'Homme et des Vertébrés (French translation by L. Azoulay) Maloine Paris, 1909–1911. The description of the discovery of the Golgi method does not appear in the original Spanish edition Textura del sistema nervioso del Hombre y de los vertebrados, Moya Madrid (1899–1904), to which we refer mainly in this article. Most of the English translation of this beautiful passage of Cajal has been taken from an article by S.L. Palay and V. Chan Palay: Cell form as an expression of neuron function, published in Golgi centennial symposium, M. Santini ed, Raven Press, New York, 1975, pp 51–60. We are indebted to Prof. S.L. Palay for providing us with a complete translation.
2. Golgi C. Sulla struttura della sostanza grigia del cervello. Gazzetta Medica Italiana (Lombardia) 1873; 6: 244–6.
3. Ramón y Cajal S. (1923) Recuerdos de mi vida. (3a ed.) Pueyo, Madrid (English translation by E. Horne Craigie and J. Cano in Recollections of my Life, published in 1937, as Memoirs of American Philosophical Society, Philadelphia).
4. Ramón y Cajal S. Estructura de los centros nerviosos de las aves. Rev Trim Histol Normal Patol 1888; 1: 1–10. (Republished in Trabajos escogidos, Vol. 1, pp. 305–315, Jménez y Molina, Madrid 1924).
5. Ramón y Cajal S. Sobre las fibras nerviosas de la capa molecular del cerebelo. Rev Trim Histol Normal Patol 1888; 2. (Republished in Trabajos escogidos, vol. 1, pp. 343–353, Jménez y Molina, Madrid 1924).
6. Ramón y Cajal S. Morphologia y conexiones de los elementos de la retina de las aves. Rev Trim Histol Normal Patol 1888; 1: 11–16. (Republished in Trabajos escogidos, Vol. 1, pp.

317–322, Jmenez y Molina, Madrid 1924).
7. Ramón y Cajal S. Estructura de la retina de las aves. Rev Trim Histol Normal Patol 1888; 2. (Republished nel 1924 in "Trabajos escogidos", Vol. 1, pp. 355–371., Jmenez y Molina, Madrid 1924).
8. Gerlach J. Von dem Rückenmarke. In: Stricker S. Handbuch der Lehre von den Geweben, pp. 665–693. Engelmann, Lipsia, 1871.
9. Golgi C. Sulla fina anatomia degli organi centrali del sistema nervoso. Riv Sper Feniatria tomi VIII–XI, 1882–1885. (also published as a book in 1886 by Hoepli, Milano).
10. Cimino G. La mente e il suo substratum. Pisa: Domus Galileiana, 1984.
11. Flourens P. Recherches expérimentales sur les propriétés et fonctions du système nerveux dans les animaux vertébrés. 1st ed., Crévot, Paris, 1828; 2nd ed., Ballière, Paris, 1842.
12. Golgi C. La rete nervosa diffusa degli organi centrali del sistema nervoso. Suo significato fisiologico. (R. Ist. Lomb. Scienze e Lettere, XXIV: Republished in French in Arch Ital Biol 1891; 15: 434–463).
13. Goltz FL. Der Hund ohne Grosshirn. Pflüg Arch ges Physiol 1892; 51; 570–614.
14. His W. Zur Geschichte des menschlichen Rückenmarkes und der Nervenwurzeln. Abh math phys Classe Sächs Gesell Wiss 1886; 13: 457–514.
15. Forel AH. Einige hirnanatomische Betrachtungen und Ergebnisse. Arch Psych Nervenkrank 1887; 18: 162–198.
16. Ramón y Cajal S. La rétine des Vertébrés. La Cellule 1893; 9: 119–257.
17. Ramón y Cajal S. Le réticule neurofibrillaire dans la rétine Trab Lab Inv Biol Univ Madrid 1901; 1: 151–157.
18. Ramón y Cajal S. Sur la morphologie et les connexions des éléments de la rétine des oiseaux. Anat Anz 4 1889; 4: 111–121.
19. Ramón y Cajal S. Nouvelles contributions à l'étude histologique de la rétine. J Anatom Physiol (Paris) 1896; 32: 480–543.
20. Waldeyer, W. Ueber einige neuere Forschungen im Gebiete der Anatomie des Centralnervensystems. V. Deutsche Med Wochenzeitschr 1891; 1352–1356.
21. Ramón y Cajal S. Communication presented at the "Congreso Médico de Valencia", published in Revista de Ciencias Médicas de Barcelona 1891; pp. 1–15.
22. Thorpe SA, Glickstein M. Introduction to: The Structure of the Retina, C. Thomas, Springfield , 1972. (English edition of the La rétina des Vertébrés, ref. 16).
23. Sterling P Microcircuitry of the cat retina. Ann Rev Neurosci 1983; 6; 149–185.
24. Kolb H, Nelson R. Neural architecture of the cat retina. Progr Retinal Res 1984; 3: 21–60.
25. Tartuferi F. Sulla anatomia della retina. Arch Sci Med 1887; 11: 335–358.
26. Embden G. Primitivfibrillenverlauf in der Netzhaut Arch f mikrosk Anat 1901; 57: 570–593.
27. Bennett MVL, Spray DC, eds. "Gap junctions" Cold Spring Harbor Press, 1984.
28. Piccolino M, Neyton J, Gerschenfeld HM. Decrease of gap junction permeability induced by dopamine and cyclic adenosine 3′:5′-monophosphate in horizontal cells of the turtle retina. J Neurosci 1984; 4: 2477–88.
29. Piccolino M, Witkovsky P, Trimarchi C. Dopaminergic mechanism underlying the reduction of electrical coupling between horizontal cells of the turtle retina induced by D-amphetamine, bicuculline and veratridine. J Neurosci 1987; 7: 2273–2284.
30. Piccolino M, Witkovsky P. Local circuits in the distal retina of the vertebrates. In Comparative Physiology of Sensory Mechanisms. L Bolis, RD Keynes, S Maddrell eds., 1984, pp. 371–404. Cambridge University Press, Cambridge.
31. Piccolino M, Trimarchi C. Lateral interactions between vertebrate photoreceptors. Photoch Photobiol 1987; 45: 305–314.
32. Stell WK. The morphological organization of the vertebrate retina. In: Fuortes MGF (ed.): Physiology of Photoreceptor Organs, pp. 11–213, 1972, Springer, Berlin.

33. Stell WK. Horizontal cell axons and axon terminals in goldfish retina. J Comp Neurol 1975; 169: 503–520.
34. Schiefferdecker P. Studien zur vergleichenden Histologie der Retina. Arch f mikrosk Anat 1886; 28: 305–396.
35. Ramón y Cajal S. Les problèmes histophysiologiques de la rétine. XIV Conc Ophthal Hispan 1933; 11: 11–19.
36. Ramón y Cajal S. Significación próbable de las células nerviosas de cilindro-eje corto. Trab Lab Inv Biol Univ Madrid 1901; 1: 151–157.
37. Ratliff F. Mach Bands: Quantitative studies on neural network in the retina. Holden-Day, San Francisco, 1965.
38. Baylor DA, Fuortes MGF, O'Bryan PM. Receptive field of cones in the retina of the turtle. J Physiol 1971; 214: 265–294.
39. Sherrington CS. The Integrative Action of the Nervous System, Constable, London, 1906.
40. Sherrington CS. Santiago Ramón y Cajal 1852–1934. Obituary Notice of the Roy Soc of London 1935; n. 4: 425–441.
41. Apathy S. Das leitende Element des Nervensystems und seine topographischen Beziehungen zu den Zellen. Mitt Zool Stat Neapel, 1897.
42. Bethe A. Allgemeine Anatomie und Physiologie des Nervensystems. Leipzig: Thieme, 1903.
43. Ramón y Cajal S. Les preuves objectives de l'unité anatomique des cellules nerveuses. Trav Lab Rech Biol Univ Madrid 1934; 29: 1–137 (English translation by MU Purkiss and CA Fox in Neuron theory or reticular theory? The objective evidence of the anatomical unity of nerve cells, CSIC, Madrid, 1954).
44. Luciani L. Fisiologia dell'Uomo. S.E.L. Milano 1905.
45. Tello JF. Santiago Ramón y Cajal: sa formation et son oeuvre. Trav Lab Rech Biol Univ Madrid 30: 1–210.

Address for correspondence: M. Piccolino, Istituto di Neurofisiologia del C.N.R., via S. Zeno 51, I-56100, Pisa, Italy.

Documenta Ophthalmologica 71: 143–154, 1989.

On the 700th anniversary of the death of Ibn an-Nafis (b. ca. 1210, d. 1288)

N. HAMARNEH
University of Damascus, Syria

Introduction

In 1924, a medical thesis [1] appeared in Germany and caused a real sensation among medical historians in Europe. Its author was Dr Muhyi āl-Dīn al-Tatāwī. While preparing for his thesis, he accidentally came across one of Ibn an-Nafīs' works in the Berlin Royal Library. He found the manuscript so informative that he decided to delve more deeply into it. What he found there induced him to base his dissertation on the works of this scientist. His discovery really surprised Europeans: Ibn an-Nafīs was the first author in history to describe the pulmonary circulation.

Why did this news surprise European medical historians?

After all Ibn an-Nafīs was not unknown:

In the Orient, for instance, he was highly regarded. His name was included in all biographies dealing with authors, outstanding men and "learned men of theology". Many commentaries on his works had been written up to the early 20th century. He was especially known through his work *Al-Mūjiz fi'l-tibb* (The Epitome of Medicine). In India this work and many commentaries on it were published again and again.

In Europe, however, things were different. It was common knowledge for scholars that most libraries there kept various works of Ibn an-Nafīs. Those available in Berlin's Royal Library, for example, had, like all Arabic manuscripts there, been described by W. Ahlwardt in his Catalogue of Arabic Manuscripts [2].

Why were the findings contained in Dr Tatāwī's thesis so sensational and almost incredible to experts in Europe? The reason is simple. No one seemed to have seriously studied Ibn an-Nafīs' works. Therefore, neither his quality as an author (as regards the general contents, the arrangement of chapters etc.), nor his scientific message (the exact facts and ideas he conveyed in the chapters) had been recognized properly.

The surprise caused by the sudden discovery of the scientific contents of a single chapter of one of Ibn an-Nafīs' books was a clear indication that neither the great achievements of this scientist nor the real importance of the

Islamic–Arabic epoch represented by him had been comprehended in Europe. Indeed, it overturned the belief held in Europe for centuries that the classical Greek period was followed by the dark Middle Ages and that there was no creative activity until the Renaissance, especially in the field of medicine.

Experts in Europe were therefore little prepared to accept the great achievements of the Islamic–Arabic epoch [3].

Dark Middle Ages or a Golden Age of science?

European historians of science often refer to the period stretching from the 9th to the 12th centuries as the dark Middle Ages. Yet, does this description hold true for that epoch in all parts of the world? As far as Latin (Western) Europe is concerned, it applies fully. Here, the medieval period was marked by a clear decline of science.

But what was going on at the same time in the East was quite the opposite. In that part of the world the contributions of the Greeks were studied and further developed. The Greeks preserved, enriched and further developed the sciences originating in earlier civilizations (Egyptian, Mesopotamian), thus raising the cultivation of science to a high level that was maintained in the Hellenistic epoch by themselves and the people of the Orient alike.

When the Roman Empire was finally split into a Western and Eastern part, the tradition of carefully cultivating science continued in the Hellenistic sense in Byzantium and in the Orient, a development that also continued with the emergence of Islam. The different nations united in the Islamic Empire (stretching from Spain via Northern Africa, Central Asia and Northern India up to the border of China) upheld that tradition by further developing science.

One can arrive at the conclusion that while Europe was going through the dark Middle Ages, the Orient experienced a true Golden Age in the cultivation of science [4].

It can justifiably be said that the Renaissance in Europe did not emerge from nothing, but was the result of the normal development of science, coming from the Islamic Orient, passing through Southern Italy and Spain and finally reaching Western and Central Europe.

Unfortunately, many historians of science in Europe did not understand this development. They were not able to expect contributions from a person living in the Arabic world in the period of the Middle Ages.

Even today, the Islamic–Arabic period in the history of culture and science is still neglected. A good example is Ibn an-Nafīs whose works are available everywhere but have not yet been carefully studied. We still do not know the extent of his contributions.

In addition, Ibn an-Nafīs is just one example of a large number of scientists of his epoch.

In this article we want to make a modest commemoration of the 700th anniversary of Ibn an-Nafīs' death. There are two important fields which we will not deal with here, but want to leave for later publication: First, a comparison of newly discovered manuscripts of his work *On Ophthalmology* and, second, his achievements in this field, particularly his contributions to the theory of vision and the pathology of eye diseases.

The life of Ibn an-Nafīs

There is little known about the life of Ibn an-Nafīs. He was born around 1210 in a small village near Damascus, called "al-Qurashi¯yah", for which reason many Arab authors and biographers also refer to him as al-Qurashī. He began his study of medicine in Damascus and received his practical medical training at the famous Nurī Hospital. Among the students of his renowned teacher al-Dakhwār was Ibn abī Usaibi [c]ah, another contemporary who became famous as a great medical historian and biographer. Besides medicine, Ibn an-Nafīs studied grammar, logic and Islamic theology.

After completing his medical studies, Ibn an-Nafīs left Damascus and went to practise medicine in Cairo which was another centre of the Arabic State. There, he became Chief Physician of Egypt and the personal physician of Sultan al-Malik al-Zāhir Baybars, one of the most important rulers of the Mamluk State, who reigned from 1260 to 1277. In Cairo, Ibn an-Nafīs practised medicine, especially ophthalmology, trained a number of students and gave lectures on law at the "al-Masrūriyya" Faculty of Theology. He became very rich and a man of great influence. He died in Cairo on 18th December 1288 at the age of about 80 years, leaving his house and library to the Cairo Mansūrī Hospital.

Ibn an-Nafīs became very prominent and popular as a learned man. He was consulted by a large number of scholars and students who visited him in his luxurious house for talks and discussions. He was considered a great practical physician, at the same time even more as an important theorist who became famous as one of the great figures in the fields of Islamic law, jurisprudence, theology and medicine. He was a prolific author of many medical works and commentaries on Greek physicians, notably on Hippocrates.

Ibn an-Nafīs: the commentator

In general, the literary activity of Ibn an-Nafīs both as a commentator and author was extensive, covering a wide range of various topics. As is evident from what he has written, Ibn an-Nafīs was a real polymath whose interests went far beyond his special domain, ophthalmology, and even medicine in general. He delved into a wide range of sciences, dealing with Arabic language, grammar and rhetoric, logic and philosophy. We can mention here his well known works on the science of Islamic tradition, in which he investigated specifically jurisprudence (fiqh) and Islamic law (sharīʿa). He also wrote on logic as a summary of Aristotle's "Organon and Rhetoric".

His *al-Risālā al-Kāmiliyyā fi 'l-sīrā al-nabawiyyā* (on Islamic philosophy and theology) [5] is regarded as one of his most important works, in which he shows his abilities as a philosopher, theologian and historian of Islam.

Beginning with the 14th century, Ibn an-Nafīs received the recognition of a large number of biographers, the two most important ones being al-Safadī (d. 1333) and al-ʿumarī (d. 1348) [6].

He wrote commentaries on Hippocrates' works *Prognostics*, *Epidemics*, *De natura hominis* and *Aphorisms*, which became especially well known. Furthermore he is the author of a commentary on Hunain ibn Ishāq's *al-Masā'lil fi l-tib* (Questions of Medicine). He also wrote *Sharh al-Qānūn*, as well as *Mūjīz al-Qānūn* (The Epitome of Medicine), a summary of this work. The latter two writings deserve special explanation.

The commentary on Ibn-Sīnā

In the commentary, *Sharh al-Qānūn*, consisting of four books (instead of five as in Ibn-Sīna's original work), Ibn an-Nafīs was critical of the order of presentation of the subject-matter in Ibn-Sīnā's *Kītāb al-Qānūn*. Ibn an-Nafīs' Book I contains two parts: (1) *Sharh Kullīyāt al-Qānūn* (Commentary on the Generalities) and (2) *Sharh Tashrīh al-Qānūn* (Commentary on the Anatomy).

The first one deals with the following topics: (i) theory of medicine: elements, qualities, humors, spirits etc.; (ii) physiology; (iii) principles of pathology, and (iv) hygiene and diet.

The second covers only anatomy. Ibn an-Nafīs placed anatomy at the end of his Book I because, as he pointed out, the topic was split up in Book I (on homogeneous organs) and Book III (on heterogeneous organs) in ibn-Sīnā's original *Kitāb al-Qānūn*.

Ibn an-Nafīs' Book I became extremely popular and was later often republished under the title *Sharh al-Kullīyāt*, leaving out the part on anatomy, which was reissued as a separate volume entitled *Sharh al-Tashrīh* (Commentary on Anatomy). In it, Ibn an-Nafīs presented his own theory of blood circulation, correcting the ideas of Galen and Ibn-Sīnā [7].

In his Book II, Ibn an-Nafīs deals with "materia medica" and complex drugs, combining Books II and V of Ibn-Sīnā's *al-Qānūn*.

In Book III, he describes "Diseases of the Body" (according to organs), and in Book IV "Diseases of General Nature", such as fevers, swellings, ulcers, poisonings, plagues and injuries, as well as bone setting and dermatology.

The Epitome of Medicine

The above-mentioned summary of *al-Qānūn* (The Epitome of Medicine) was published under the titles *Mūjiz al-Qānūn* or *al-Mūjīz* as a practical handbook. It was also very popular, and later several commentaries were written on it [8].

Ibn an Nafīs: the author

As an author, Ibn an-Nafīs won fame for himself due to several works of which the three major ones are mentioned here: The first one was a handbook and quick reference for students and practitioners, describing aetiology, symptomatology and treatment of diseases in the form of a very short summary [9].

Probably Ibn an-Nafīs' last work is *Kitab al-Shāmil fi'l Sināʿa al-tibbiyya*, a "Comprehensive Book on the Art of Medicine". He had planned to write 300 volumes, yet could complete only 80 before his death, of which at least ten are known today.

The third book called *al-Muhaddab* (The Perfected Book) deals with Ibn an-Nafīs' special domain, ophthalmology, and shall, therefore, be examined more in detail at the end of this article.

The lesser circulation

Ibn an-Nafīs exerted a tremendous influence on his contemporaries and the generations after him. Suffice it to mention two authors from the orient who wrote two well known commentaries on Ibn-Sina's *al-Qānūn*, published in 1344 by Sadīd ad-Dīn al-Kāzarūnī and in 1350 by Zayn al-ʿArab al-Misrī [10]. Both of them adopted, preserved and defended Ibn an-Nafīs' theory of pulmonary circulation.

Other authors did not recognize the great contribution made by Ibn an-Nafīs to physiology. Some of them simply did not know about it, while others were well aware of it but neglected and ignored it.

But there even was at least one who rejected Ibn an-Nafīs' views and defended Galen and Ibn-Sīnā [11].

A successor who merits comment is Andrea Alpago who lived in the 15th and early 16th c. He translated some of Ibn an-Nafīs' works into Latin, which were later printed in Padua, Italy. It is likely that Servetus and Colombo came across some of Alpago's translations and thus became acquainted with Ibn an-Nafīs' theory of pulmonary circulation [12].

Ibn an Nafīs was fully aware of his fundamental opposition to Galen's viewpoint on anatomy and physiology. At least three points on which he opposed Galen are [13].

"1. Galen's *movement* of the blood is replaced by Ibn an-Nafīs' *blood circulation.*

"2. *The interventricular septum is non-porous*, and contrary to the opinions of Galen and others, it has no visible or invisible pores.

"3. Galen's aeration of the blood in the left ventricle is unacceptable to Ibn an-Nafīs who says that the blood must pass from the right ventricle through the pulmonary artery into the lungs where it is aerated, and back from the lungs into the pulmonary vein to the left ventricle."

Ibn an-Nafīs was conscious of the importance of his correction of Galen. He wrote in his introductory note to his *Sharh K. al-Qānūn* (Commentary on Anatomy), among other things, that he was going to "explain all queries and clarify all doctrines ... and stand by true opinions, and forsake those which are false and erase their traces" [14].

The Perfected Book on Ophthalmology *(Al-Muhaḏḏab)*

The *Perfected Book on Opthalmology* consists of a preface and two main parts.

The preface is divided into three chapters one of which is important because it contains a comparative anatomy of the eyes of some animals, influenced by Aristotle.

In general, the first part deals with the *principles* of ophthalmology from a theoretical point of view, while the second part delves into the *details* of the science.

The first main part is composed of two sections. The first section dealing with the principles of the *theoretical* aspects of ophthalmology has four

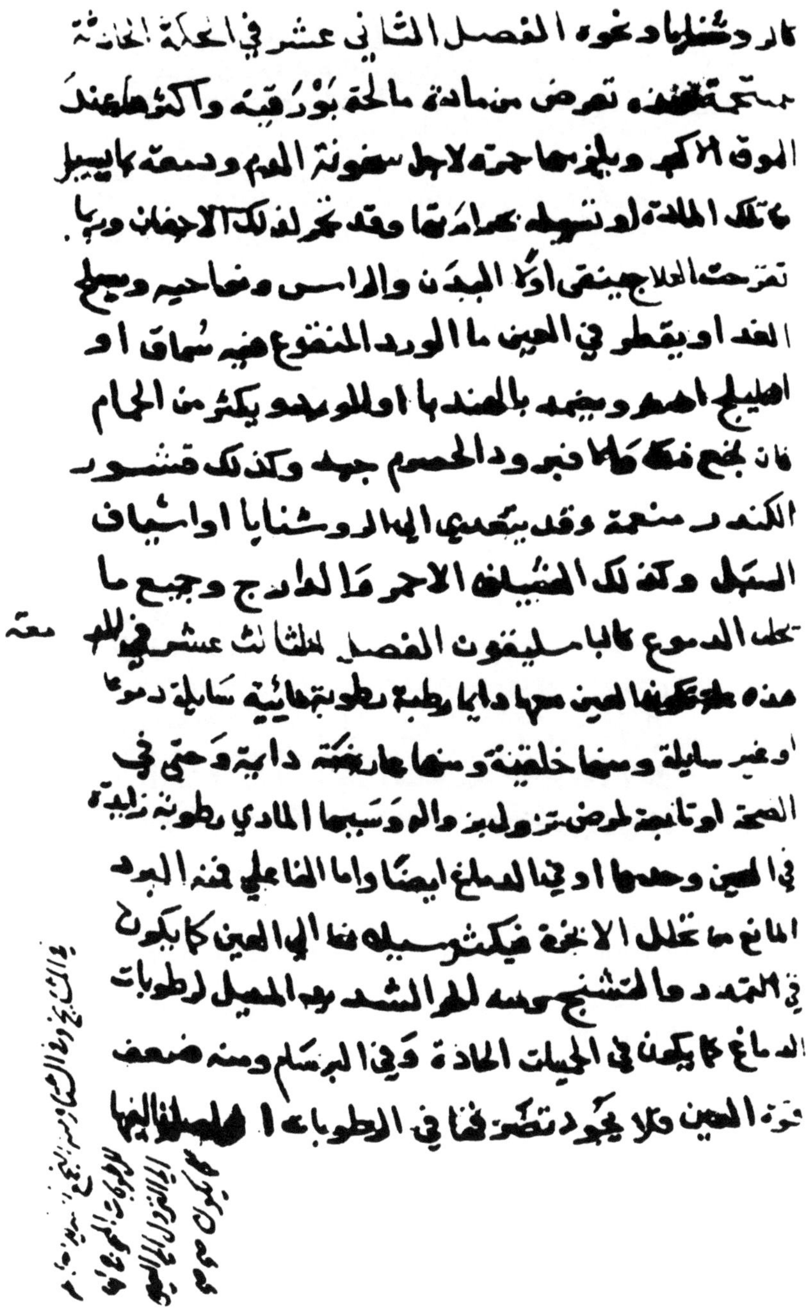

Fig. 1. (AL-MUHADDAB) Manuscript Berlin or. oct. 2365. Revealed for the first time by Rudolf Sellheim in: Materialien zur arabischen Literaturgeschichte. (Verzeichniß der orientalischen Handschriften in Deutschland XVIII, A.) Wiesbaden: Steiner 1976, pp. 213–216.

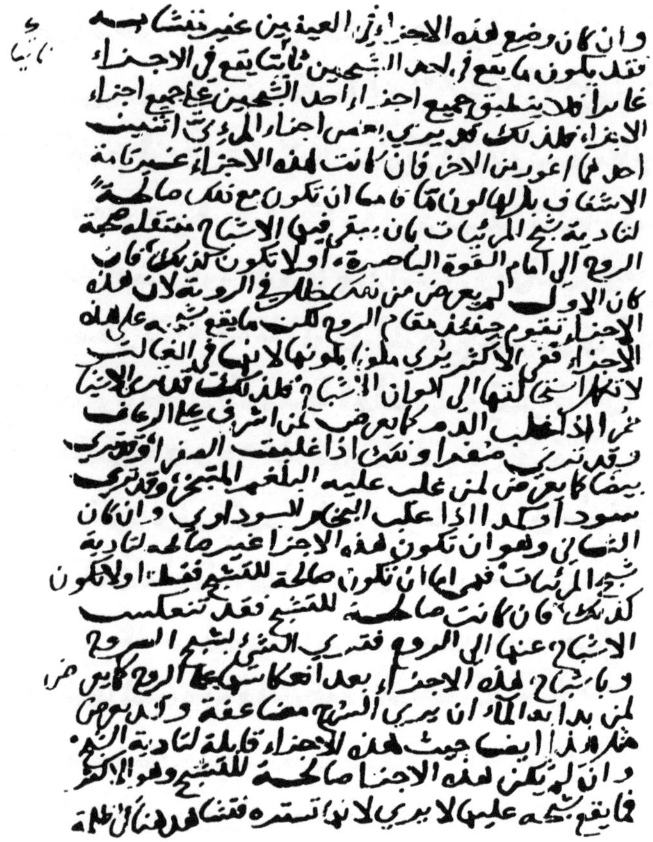

Fig. 2. (AL-MUHADDAB) Manuscript Damascus Zāhirīya 8435. For the first time presented to the public by Dr Schammut (Damascus) in: Supreme Council of Sciences (Year Book – 1967).

cf. N. Hamarneh, First Reading in a 13th Century Manuscript in Ophthalmology Written by Ibn an-Nafīs. Aleppo, 1978.

cf. also S. Khiami, Index of Manuscripts on Medicine, Pharmacy and Allied Sciences in the Zāhirīya Library, Vol. II. Damascus, 1981.

divisions: (1) anatomy and physiology; (2) pathology; (3) aetiology; and (4) symptomatology.

The second section considers the principles of *practical* ophthalmology in two divisions: (1) the hygiene of the eye; and (2) general management and treatment.

Each of the divisions is subdivided into various chapters.

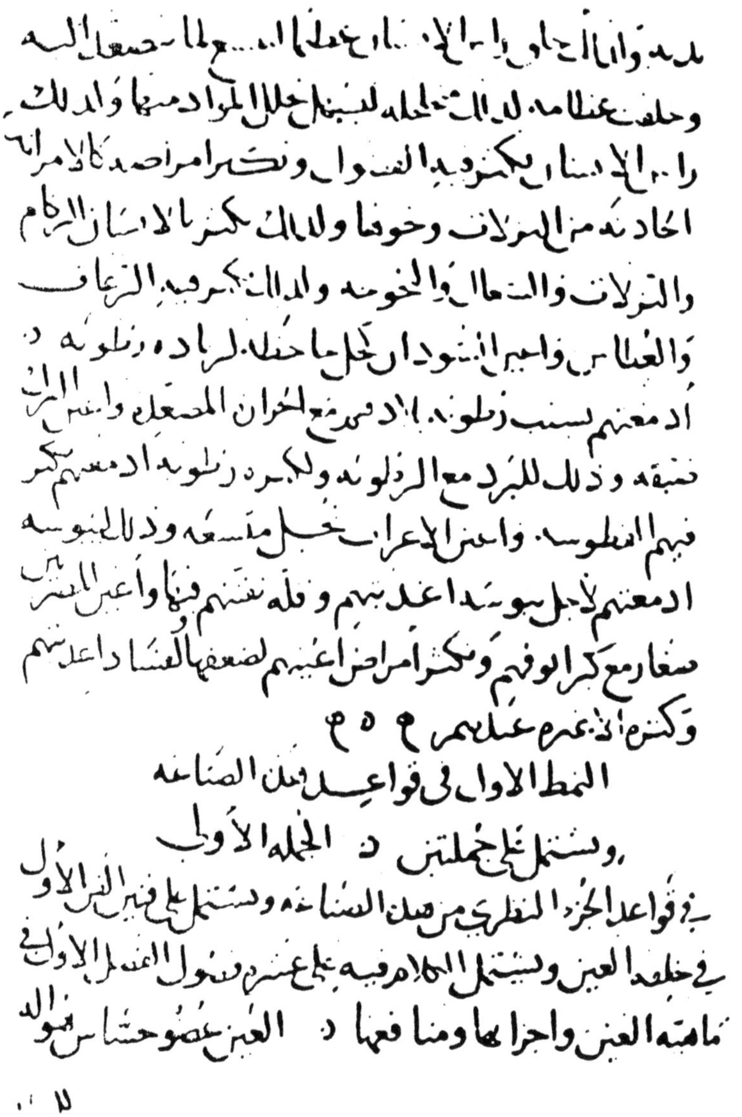

النمط الاول في قواعد علم الصناعة

ويشتمل على جملتين الجملة الاولى

Fig. 3. (AL-MUHADDAB) Manuscript Istanbul – H. Mahmud 5515.
cf. F. Sezgin, Geschichte des arabischen Schrifttums, Vol. III. Leiden, 1970, p. 339.

For the first time identified and revealed to the scientific community by the author *s.* Nashaat Hamarneh, The Ophthalmology of Ibn an-Nafīs (The Perfected Book on Ophthalmology)(Al-Muhaddab fī l-kuhl) in: Supreme Council of Sciences. Damascus, 1981 (Year Book – 1981).

The second main part. of the *Perfected Book on Ophthalmology* consists of seven sections.

The first section deals with ocular remedies, examining in its first division "practical principles" and in its second division "principles of ocular drugs" which are dealt with in two chapters on "simple drugs" and "complex drugs".

The second section considers diseases of the *external* parts (*the adnexi*) of the eye. The first of its two divisions deals with *eye-lids* and has 30 chapters, each of them examining one of the diseases of the eye-lids, while the second division (containing three chapters) describes diseases of the *lacrimal* system.

The third section focuses on diseases of the *middle* part of the eye-ball. It has four divisions, each of them divided into chapters covering a specific disease:

1. diseases of the *conjunctiva* (13 chapters),
2. diseases of the *cornea* (7 chapters)
3. diseases of the *iris and the ciliary body* (3 chapters),
4. diseases related to the *pupil* (3 chapters).

The fourth section considers diseases of the *eye-ball* as a whole, which are described in three chapters: (1) *Strabismus*; (2) *Exophthalmus*; (3) *Enophthalmus*.

The fifth section consists of seven chapters examining problems of *visual acuity*.

The sixth section takes into account "diseases of the *humors* and *spirits* of the eye".

The seventh section deals with diseases of other parts of the eye in two chapters the first of which concentrates *on layers* of the eye and the second on the *optic nerve*.

Examining the *Perfected Book on Ophthalmology* today, the reader will become aware that Ibn an-Nafīs was not only a first-rank theorist, but also an outstanding practitioner and eye surgeon.

If the reader is a physician or an ophthalmologist, he will admire Ibn an-Nafīs' great accuracy in describing clinical pictures and thanks to these brilliant descriptions will be able to imagine the manifestations of diseases in such a lively manner as if he were reading a patient's clinical record or examining the patient himself.

As far as eye surgery is concerned, the modern reader will admire Ibn an-Nafīs' ability as a surgeon and his descriptions of the smallest details of the various kinds of surgical techniques. He even described certain changes he made in surgical instruments resulting from his wide practical knowledge acquired over many years of work.

He was so convinced from his ophthalmological experience that he even rejected some theories on the pathology of eye diseases, replacing them by his own.

For all these reasons, the 700th anniversary of Ibn an-Nafīs' death should be an appropriate occasion for physicians in general and ophthalmologists in particular to learn about his life and work and to become acquainted with the great store of knowledge he bequeathed to his contemporaries, and to future generations.

Ibn an-Nafīs was one of many great men who made original contributions to the development of ophthalmology. Furthermore, he is one of the major authors in the history of ophthalmology.

Therefore we should honour the memory of Ibn an-Nafīs, a remarkable polymath, great physician and outstanding ophthalmologist.

Notes

1. Muhyī āl Dīn al Tatāwi¯, *Der Lungenkreislauf nach el-Koraschi*, mimeographed thesis, Freiburg i. Br., 1924.
2. W. Ahlwardt, *Verzeichniß der arabischen Handschriften der Königlichen Bibliothek zu Berlin*, 10 Bde, Berlin 1887–1899.
3. In addition, there was another deeply rooted and widespread idea among European historians of science, including medical historians: They believed that the beginnings of medicine and the sciences in general were to be sought in Greek Antiquity. They therefore neglected a study of the origins of Greek medicine. These historians ignored that the Greeks themselves had expressly admitted that they had taken over much of the materia medica from Egypt.
4. This point of view was represented by Julius Hirschberg who stated in *The History of Ophthalmology*: "Thus the Arabs carefully tended and maintained the flame of science in the first half of the Middle Ages, i.e. from the eighth to the twelfth centuries, at a time when it had almost completely gone out in Europe."
   (Die Araber haben also in der ersten Hälfte des Mittelalters, vom achten bis zum zwölften Jahrhundert, die Flamme der Wissenschaft sorgsam gepflegt und unterhalten, zu einer Zeit, wo sie in Europa fast ganz erloschen war.)
   In: Julius Hirschberg, *Geschichte der Augenheilkunde*, Zweites Buch, Leipzig, 1908, p. 4.
5. See M. Meyerhof and J. Schacht, *The theologus autodidactus of Ibn an-Nafīs*, Oxford, 1968.
6. Other successors who in the 14th century highly praised his life, influence and important work were
   - al-Dhahabī (d. 1348,
   - al-Subkī (d. 1370), and
   - al-Yafiʿī (d. 1376).

   Later on, all biographers appreciated him as a very important authority.
7. See Max Meyerhof, *Ibn al-Nafīs und seine Theorie des Lungenkreislaufs*, in: Quellen und Studien zur Geschichte der Naturwissenschaften und der Medizin, iv, Berlin, 1935, pp. 37–88.
8. The major commentators on al-Mūjiz were

- al-Suwaidī (died towards the end of the 13th century,
- al-Kāzarūnī (d. in the middle of the 14th c.),
- al-Aqsarā'ī (d. towards the end of the 14th c.),
- al-Kirmānī (d. in the middle of the 15th c.), and
- al-Amshātī (living in the 15th c.).

9. The original title of the handbook is: *Bugyat at-Talibīn wa Hğğat al-Mutatabbibīn.*
10. See A.Z. Iskander, *A catalogue of Arabic manuscripts on medicine and science in the Wellcome Historical Medical Library*, London, 1967, pp. 181–183.
11. al-Fādil al-Bagghdādī (lived after the 14th century). Manuscript Berlin We. 1187 (see Ahlwardt 6294, p. 556).
12. See Meyerhof and Schacht in the "Encyclopaedia of Islam" (2nd ed., vol. III, p. 898): "A theory of the lesser circulation, identical in all essential respects with that of Ibn an-Nafīs and expressed in terms strangely reminiscent of those used by him, was formulated by Michael Servetus in his *Christianismi restitutio* (Vienna 1553), and an exposition of the same doctrine by Realdus Columbus (Realdo Colombo) in his *De re anatomica libri XV* (Venice 1559) forms a close parallel to this. Detailed philological analysis has made it probable that Servetus (and perhaps Colombo, too) had direct knowledge of the theory of Ibn an-Nafīs, and it is likely that this knowledge was transmitted by Andrea Alpago, who spent more than 30 years in Syria, travelled widely in search of Arabic manuscripts, and is known to have translated from the Arabic numerous medical texts not all of which were printed posthumously (he died about 1520)."
13. Summarized by Prof. Iskander. (Personal communication).
14. Prof. A.Z. Iskander has translated this introductory note of which we publish the following excerpt: "We shall explain all queries and clarify all doctrines, except those which are frivolous and are wanting of intelligence. We shall present our investigations in an orderly way, and shall carefully discuss and consider them until we are able to shed light on and stand by true opinions, and forsake those which are false and erase their traces. But should declaration of the truth about certain doctrines require investigations in matters irrelevant to this book, we would have to rely on, (and refer to), our simplified books. Our investigations in theory may lead us to forsake familiar and commonplace knowledge: what reaches the ear will be different from the well-known! But we shall not rashly deny anything; this would tantamount to recklessness. Perhaps a (doctrine) to which men adhere is genuine, yet another familiar one is false. For the truth, in reality, is true; not on account of what people say. Let us remember their statement: 'If people's intellects and endeavours are equal, then – in all arts – the successors are superior to their predecessors.'"

Address for correspondence: N. Hamarneh, Dolgenseestr. 55, Berlin 1136, GDR.

Documenta Ophthalmologica 71: 155–165, 1989.

The treatment of eye diseases in the Asclepieia

S. MARKETOS, J.N. FRONIMOPOULOS & J. LASKARATOS
National University of Athens, School of Medicine, Department of History of Medicine, Athens, Greece

Abstract. The authors give a short report of ophthalmic treatment in Asclepieia by the priests, who had learned these cures through tradition from other priests.

This can be testified by the writings on the stone tablets, which were found in the excavations of the Asclepieion at Epidaurus (1883). They give information concerning illnesses and their treatment.

From this historical source we selected certain cases with eye-diseases and their treatment. Included is a part from Aristophanes' comedy "Ploutos", giving interesting ophthalmic treatments.

These treatments by the priests, representing God Asclepius, mainly took the form of medicines and operations performed in a psychologically mysterious atmosphere.

The treatment of eye diseases in the Asclepieia is a historical fact, confirmed by bibliographic studies in old and recent papers. From the various references in these and similar publications, we selected information, which after classification, we found interesting enough to make this short account of.

It is well known that Asclepius was an eminent doctor in the pre-Homeric period, as well as being sovereign of Triki and Ithomi, and father of two eminent doctors, Machaon and Podalirios, who participated in the Trojan war. During the 6th century B.C., he was proclaimed a god, and the temples dedicated to him in the next ten centuries developed into famous hospitals, where besides his adoration, medical care was offered by the priests.

The temples were established in specially selected places, in order to offer – apart from the treatment – a naturally healthy environment to patients, thus helping their recovery.

The establishment of the Asclepieia as therapeutic centres occurred at the end of the 6th century B.C., and the adoration of the new god, which started at Epidaurus, spread quickly and continued until the 5th century A.D. Of these temples, about 400 are known. Among them are the Asclepieia of Trikis, Tithorea of Fokis, Epidaurus, Milos, Cos, Rhodes, Piraeus, Argos, Leuctra and Sparta.

Attached to these temples, were institutions for the entertainment of the patients and their accompanying relatives, such as theatres, conservatories, etc. (Fronimopoulos & Lambrou, 1981).

Patients treated there were not only uneducated, credulous people, but also outstanding personalities and leaders of the ancient culture, such as the philosopher Crantor, the orators Eschinis and Aristides, the comedian Theopombos and many others mentioned by recent historians, Kavadias (1884, 1891, 1900), Aravantinos (1907), Zervos (1914), Koysis (1929), Georgiou (1972), Bettmann (1979) and others.

Although the total number of treatments used in these holy institutions is unknown, we have found some elements and facts about the divine medical, pharmaceutical or surgical cures effected by the priest doctors, representing the god at night while the patients were asleep.

The archeologist Kavadias (1884, 1891, 1900), believed that in the Asclepieia, patients were submitted to pharmaceutical treatment, which at that time was a popular and practical art. Thus the treatment in the temples was based mainly on holy faith and on the credulity and superstition of the patients. Kavadias considered that the healing of the blind, the lame and other incurable cases recorded on the stone tablets found during excavation of these temples, were not entirely true, but an exaggeration of the treatment and healing effects.

However, it seems that in reality medicines were used and operations were performed on patients in the temples, in combination with physical training, hygienic nourishment, sport and entertainment. The treatments were effected by the priests, who had learned the cures through tradition and the holy art of Asclepius from older priests. They performed these cures under the mantle of divine dependance and inspiration. People accepted the whole procedure, as they believed in the divine origin of the diseases, and that only a holy force could cure them.

All this can be testified by the writings on the stone tablets, mentioned by the historians Pausanias and Stravon, which were found in the excavations of the Asclepieion at Epidaurus, 1883. On these stone tablets was found information about the illnesses and their treatment, somewhat like today's medical records; it was also found that many patients suffering from eye diseases went to the temple seeking to be treated by the god.

From all the literature we studied concerning the stone tablets, we have selected certain cases where eye-diseases were treated. The cases that follow are based on personal translations (Laskaratos 1980) of old texts taken from stone tablets selected by the archeologist Kavadias (1884, 1891, 1900) and from the works of Baunack (1890) and Reinach (1884).

Case No. 1

Ambrosia of Athens was one-eyed. She came to pray to the god. Walking

> through the temple, she laughed at certain treatments, believing it impossible for the blind and lame to be cured through mere dreams. However, when she fell asleep she dreamed that the god appeared and said that she would be cured, but that she should offer, as a dedication to the temple, a silver pig, as a reminder of her thoughtlessness. After the god had said all this, he opened her lids and poured a certain medicine onto the sick eye. Soon after day-break she left, cured.

In discussing this cure and the way it was performed, we have to accept two significant points. Firstly, the inference that the patient had to be frightened and taught a grateful respect towards the holy cure and secondly the description of the treatment and the explanation of the kind of cure for this ophthalmic disease, effected during the patient's sleep in the holy temple by the priest, who raised the lids and administered an eye solution of unknown composition.

In this case, as in others, it should be emphasised that there is obviously a certain amount of exaggeration in the description of the cure performed.

The terminology used in the writings on the stone tablets, "one-eyed" or "blind", cannot be accepted here at face value to mean total blindness in one or both eyes, but rather a temporary obstruction of the vision due to some illness, such as simple conjunctivitis, iridocyclitis, etc., which provoke photophobia and blepharospasmus. Thus we can explain the complete cure and recovery of "blind" persons who were in fact suffering only temporary obstruction of their vision.

The short period of treatment in this case should also be considered relative. That a cure should be effected so quickly is inconceivable – even conjunctivitis cannot be cured overnight. The most probable view is that a long-term treatment was performed over several nights under repeated hypnosis. But the priest who recorded the cure on the tablet wanted to elevate the holy ability by exaggeration of the therapeutic power of the god, enabling such a rapid cure.

Case No. 2

> There came praying to the god, a one-eyed man, who, on the one side had only lids without any contents – totally empty. Thus, some of the people in the temple were discussing his stupidity in believing that he could ever see again, having no eye, but only the orbit. When he slept, he saw an apparition and thought that the god had prepared some medicine, which on raising the lids, he administered to both eyes. After day-break he left, seeing with both eyes.

There are two possible explanations in this case. Firstly, that it may have been simply an advertising cure, with the purpose of exaggerating the supernatural powers of the God in giving light to those without eyes. Secondly, that the patient had recently suffered from a disease in his one eye, healthy until that time, perhaps conjunctivitis or a swelling of the lids. The illness of the formerly healthy eye disturbed his vision. After the treatment administered to the good eye by the priest, he was cured, and left with the impression that he could see with both eyes.

The historian Aravantinos (1907) accepted the view that the patient's one eye was atrophic without vision and the other healthy. When he came out of the temple, he was able to see with his healthy eye and thought that both eyes were cured. This happened to patients suffering for many years of amblyopia or atrophy in one eye, who did not realise it until the moment they were obliged to use the non-seeing eye.

In this case it is obvious that the therapeutic remedy used was intentionally prepared by the priest in the presence of the patient. It was probably a poultice, which was placed on the good eye, which was possibly suffering from swollen lids or blepharitis, giving the patient the impression that he was blind in both eyes.

This exaggeration makes the description untrue and therefore can be regarded as being intended as an advertisement.

Case No. 3

> Alketas of Aliki who was blind had a dream. He thought he saw the god approaching him and opening with his fingers the lids of his eye. The first thing he saw were the trees in the temple park. After day-break he went out cured.

It is obvious that in this cure some operation was performed, because the god, i.e. the priest, by some manoeuvre opened the patient's lids, after which he could see again. Probably the patient had healthy eyes, but because of angyloblepharon or blepharophimosis and not blepharoptosis, his vision was hindered – an hypothesis expressed by Aravantinos (1907), difficult to accept because such conditions require complicated operations.

Again such exaggeration can only be explained as advertising.

Case No. 4

> Thison of Ermioni was a blind child, cured by a dog loitering in the temple; he left with healthy eyes.

Here again, "blindness" could be better termed "chronic disease", hindering good vision. The child was cured by having his eyes licked by trained dogs, a treatment we meet often in the Asclepieia for wounds and ulcers of the skin. The intervention of the God in this case is manifest by sending a dog, the symbol of Asclepius. The same treatment was used in the licking snakes, also symbols of Asclepius.

Case No. 5

> Hermon from Thasos was blind and cured by the god but after the treatment, the god blinded him again because he did not bring the treatment fees to the temple. When he returned and slept, the god warned him. (He probably paid the fees before entering the sanctuary this time!)

This cure does not contain any suggestion as to the kind of therapy applied and belongs to those used to frighten the bad payers, who left the temple secretly after treatment.

Case No. 6

> A man who was wounded in a battle by a spear in both eyes was blind and for one year he carried the spearhead pinned to his face. When he slept he had a dream. It seemed to him that the god pulled out the spear and applied to his lids the so called ... (a word is missing here). After daybreak he went out cured.

This cure suggests a surgical treatment. The priest moved the spear which had wounded the lids and was pinned to the face of the patient, thus hindering his vision. Here, the blindness was probably related to the lids' injuries and not to the eyes themselves. However, the injuries reported done to the lids do not denote any destruction, neither is his exit from the temple, cured, in any way related to the healthy condition of the patient's eyes but only to the removal of the spear.

Case No. 7

> Timon, who was wounded by a lance under the eye, after he slept, had a dream. He thought he saw the god, after grinding a plant, pour some of it onto the eye, and then he was cured.

Aravantinos (1907) gave the explanation that the patient must have been suffering from a traumatic inflammation after an injury to the lower lid, and was treated by the priest with an anti-inflammatory plant extract.

We think more probable the presence of a post-traumatic inflammation of the orbit, produced by a lance which had passed through under the eyeball, leaving the eye intact. This view is more probable as blindness is not mentioned in the text. The inflammation of the orbit was cured by the priest, using a plant extract.

Case No. 8

When the suppliants to the god had slept, Aeschines climbed up a tree and leaned over to see what was happening inside the sanctuary. He fell from the tree onto some sharp poles and injured his eyes badly. In a serious condition, blinded, he prayed to the god and slept. He became healthy again.

This cure was obviously designed mainly to scare people and thus discourage visitors from being curious about what happened inside the sanctuary, as well as emphasising the magnanimity of Asclepius to those who repented. There is no obvious treatment of the injuries, which Aravantinos believed must have been only superficial scratches on the lids and therefore this cure should be regarded as an exaggeration intended to stimulate the faith of the patients.

Case No. 9

Someone called Alkinoos, who was suffering in one eye was given treatment while awake.

This cure, mentioned by Aravantinos (1907), was written on part of a stone tablet and therefore, being incomplete, cannot be evaluated as to the therapeutic treatment.

Case No. 10

Alexander of Crete, who was suffering from an eye disease, was cured while asleep and payed one silver mna.

The stone tablet on which this case is written was also preserved in part only with certain phrases missing. Thus, any discussion would be purposeless and it can be accepted only as evidence of the fact that eye diseases were treated in the Asclepieia.

Case No. 11

Report of this remarkable ophthalmic cure is given to us by the ancient historian Pausanias and concerns someone called Falysios from Naupactos who was cured not in the temple, but at home. He writes:

> When Falysios was sick of an eye disease and was almost blind, the god of Epidaurus sent him the poetess Anyti with a sealed letter ... She went to Naupactos and ordered Falysios to open and read it. Falysios, although believing that he would be unable to read the letter due to the condition of his eyes, nevertheless expecting some benefit to result from the message from Asclepius, removed the seal and on looking at the wax of the seal, was cured and gave to Anyti 2000 statirs of gold, as instructed in the letter.

The kind of remedy used in this case is not mentioned and the letter was probably the bill for treatment. From Pausanias' history comes the information that Falysios founded the Asclepieion of Naupactos in gratitude to the god.

* * *

A number of clay votive offerings, discovered during excavations, testify to satisfactory numbers of patients who where treated successfully. These clay offerings are similar to silver and gold offerings, the majority of which have been stolen by plunderers during the course of time. Each offering represented a certain part of the body, which had been cured, similar to the Romans' "donaria" and dedications to the Egyptian god Isis. Among these offerings were representations of eyes, given to the temples by healed patients. Even today, similar offerings in gold or silver may be found in churches, hanging before icons.

The ancient comedian Aristophanes gives a description of the treatment of ophthalmic diseases in the Asclepieia in his comedy "Ploutos" (388 B.C.). According to Zervos (1914), Kasas & Struckmann (1979), the poet Aristophanes was himself suffering from an eye disease and was treated in the Asclepieion of Athens or Piraeus. This, of course, would explain the ease with which he describes the ophthalmic treatment of Ploutos, who had lost his vision. This work has been considered as a classic and is mentioned by many authors, such as Zervos (1914), Cousis (1929), Castiglioni (1961), Vercourte (1885, 1886). Quoted below is the part of Aristophanes' comedy which concerns the treatment in the Asclepieia:

Carion, as slave, is relating to a woman the method by which Ploutos was treated.

C. As soon as we arrived in all haste at the temple, carrying the man who until that time had been very unhappy and who is now happy and blessed above all others; we took him to the sea and gave him a bath.

W. My God! The old man must have enjoyed that – being bathed in such a cold sea!

C. Afterwards, we headed for the temple. When we had sacrificed the honey-cakes and offerings on the altar to Black Hephaestus we put Plouto to bed, as is the custom, and each of us spread out a heap of leaves.

W. Had other people come to pray to the god?

C. There was one person there, Neoclides, who, although blind, far out does the seeing where thieving is concerned! ... there were also many others suffering from various diseases. Anyway, when the priest extinguished our candles, recommending us to sleep, and telling us that even if we should hear any noise to keep quite, we all lay down. Then, afraid, I covered myself while the god walked around examining all the sick. Then, a child brought him a stone pestle and mortar and a box.

W. A stone box?

C. No, for God's sake, the box wasn't made of stone.

W. And just how did you see it, damn you, since you say you were covered?

C. By Jove, through my mantle of course, because it is full of holes. To start with, for Neoclides, he began to grind a medicine for a poultice, pounding three heads of garlic, to which he added milk from dog-onions and lentisk. After wetting the mixture with strong vinegar, he turned back the eyelids so that it would hurt even more and applied the mixture. Neoclides jumped up yelling and screaming, wanting to leave, but the god, laughingly told him to sit down covered in plaster and that in that way he would be taught not to give false oaths in the assembly.

W. How god loves the town ... and how wise he is!

C. Next, he went and sat beside Plouto. He grasped his head and with a clean towel wiped his eyelids and Panacea (the daughter of Asclepius) came and covered his head with a red cloth. Then he whistled. Immediately, two enormous snakes came out of the temple.

W. Oh, my God!

C. They slid quietly under the red cloth and started licking his lids, or so it seemed to me, and, my good woman, in less than the time it takes to drink ten glasses of wine, Plouto got up, able to see, and I clapped my hands with joy and woke up my master. And immediately both the god and the snakes disappeared into the temple. You should have seen how all those who had been lying near Plouto, embraced him and celebrated all night until day-break. I glorified the god very much, who had so quickly made Plouto see ... and who had made Neoclides even worse!

This description by Aristophanes, completes and explains further the cures written on the stone tablets found in the Epidaurus excavations. Moreover, it contains a detailed description of the preparation of a poultice, as opposed to the cases described on the stone tablets, usually reporting vaguely the treatments in order to emphasize the holy power, keeping the treatment secret, exactly as Hippocrates taught later in his law (unto holy men, holy matters).

The therapeutic work of Asclepius continued in the Roman Asclepieia, reinforced by the art of practical medicine. Remedies, baths, sport, diet and bleeding were used systematically. From stone tablets found in Rome's Asclepieion two more ophthalmic cures are known, reported by Kavadias (1900), Samothrakis (1934) and Kostomiris (1887). The first concerns the treatment of the blind man Gaios, during the reign of the Emperor Antonios. It is written:

In these days, a blind man named Gaios decided to visit the holy altar and to walk from the right to the left of the altar and place his five fingers upon it, and then raise his hand and touch his eyes and was quickly able to see. This happened in the presence of other people who were very glad that such miracles were occurring during the reign of the respected Antonios.

The second case concerns the cure of a blind soldier. The following is written on the stone table:

The god suggested to the blind soldier Valerios Aper, that he should come to the temple and take blood from a white rooster, mixed with honey and prepare a collyre, which should be administered to his eyes for three days, and he saw again, and came to thank the god publicly.

In conclusion, the stone tablets of the Epidaurus and Rome Asclepieia, and the part quoted of Aristophanes' comedy "Ploutos", give interesting descriptions of different cures and kinds of treatment. In some of them, we see an exaggeration of the god's unusual healing abilities – like miracles; in others, descriptions intended to frighten the credulous; still others may be regarded as a reminder to patients to fulfill their obligations and pay the fees for the treatment.

Thus the ophthalmic treatment in the Asclepieia, given by the priests representing the god, mainly took the form of medicines or operations under the influence of a psychologically mysterious atmosphere.

References

1. Aravantinos, A. Asclepius and the Asclepeiea. Leipzig. Defects B. Drougoulinos, 1907.
2. Baunack J, Baunack Th. Studien auf dem Gebiete des Griechischen und der Arischen Sprachen. Leipzig: Verlag von S. Hirzel, 1886.
3. Baunack J. Aus Epidaurus. Eine Epigraphische Studie. Leipzig: Verlag Von S. Hirzel, 1890.
4. Castiglioni A. History of medicine. Trans. in Greek by Papaspyroy N. Vol. 1, Athens, 1961.
5. Georgiou I. Magic-medicine. Historic review. Athens: Parisianos, 1972.
6. Bettmann LO. A pictorial history of medicine. 5th ed. Springfield, Illinois: Ch. Thomas, 1979.
7. Zervos S. The history of medicine. Vol. 1. Athens, 1914.
8. Fronimopoulos J, Lambrou N. Hippocrates and the International Hippocratic Foundation of Cos. Hist Ophth Internat 1981; 2: 157–70.
9. Kavadias P. Feuilles d'Epidaure. Athens, 1891.
10. Kavadias P. The treatment of the sick at the Asclepeion of Epidaurus. Galinos 14: 203–208, 15: 221–223, 16: 237–240, 1884.
11. Kavadias P. The sanctuary of Asclepius at Epidaurus and the treatment of the sick. Athens, 1900.
12. Kasas S, Struckmann R. Important medical centres in the Antiquity Epidaurus and Corinth. Athens, 1979.
13. Kostomiris G. About ophthalmology and otology in ancient Greece from the ancient times until Hippocrates. Athens, 1887.
14. Koyzis A. History of medicine. Athens, 1929.
15. Lascaratos J. The ophthalmological treatment in the Asclepieia. Greek Annals of Ophthalmology 1980; 17: 143–54.
16. Pausanias. Guide to Greece. "All About The Ancient Greek Writers", Papyrus, Athens, 1975.
17. Reinach Salamon. Chronique d'Orient. Revue Archeologique 1884; 4: 76–102.
18. Samothrakis A. The Greek medicine in Rome etc. Elliniki latriki 1934; 8: 1188–1203.

19. Stravonos. Geographica. "All about the Ancient Greek Writers". Papyrus, Athens, 1975.
20. Vercourte. La Médecine sacerdotale dans l'antiquité grèque. Revue Archéologique 1885; 6: 272–292, 1986; 7: 22–26, 106–123.

Address for correspondence: Prof. S. Marketos, National University of Athens, School of Medicine, Dept. of History of Medicine, Athens, Greece.

Documenta Ophthalmologica 71: 167–193, 1989.

Public health and research in the development of Russian ophthalmology

HENRY J. CARSON
Chicago, Illinois, USA

Although the Soviets display with pride the achievements of ophthalmology in the USSR [1] and routinely publish articles on ophthalmologic history in scholarly journals, little recorded in America explains how the specialty attained such eminence in Russia. George Gorin devoted two short, informative chapters in his *History of Ophthalmology* to Russian and Soviet eye doctors [2], and Anatoly Bezkorovainy published a fine review of research in late Nineteenth Century Russian ocular science [3]. Hirschberg's definitive *History of Ophthalmology* chronicles people and progress superbly in a thorough section [4]. Other information in English is scarce, however, and doesn't address the issue of how ophthalmology excelled while general medicine in Russia remained mired in a bog of inadequate resources, poorly trained personnel, and outdated therapeutics.

In her book *Russian Physicians in an Era of Reform and Revolution, 1856–1905*, Nancy Frieden provided valuable insights into the relationships between doctors, society, and state in the Russian age [5]; likewise, Mark Field's *Soviet Socialized Medicine* elucidated how these relationships changed in the Soviet era [6]. To find how ophthalmologists in particular fit into the panorama of Russian and Soviet medicine, however, required a review of historical and biographic articles and memoirs from the Soviet Press, in particular *Vestnik oftalmologii* (The Annals of Ophthalmology) and *Oftalmologicheskij zhurnal* (Ophthalmologic Journal), and a study of some important contemporary works, notably Sergei Golovin's *On Blindness in Russia* [7], Saviotov's review [8], and Filatov's *My Path in Science* [9]. While the following report isn't exhaustive, it sheds some light on ophthalmology's important place in Russian and Soviet medicine.

A brief review of ophthalmology in central Europe sets the stage for the growth of the specialty in Russia. Germany, Austria, and the Netherlands led the world in eye sciences in the Nineteenth Century. Not only did Russian doctors such as Blessig (see Fig. 1), Junge, Lozhechnikov (see Fig. 2), Braun, Ivanov, Girshman, and Pirogov study with German scholars and scientists to learn the state-of-the-art diagnosis and treatment of eye disease;

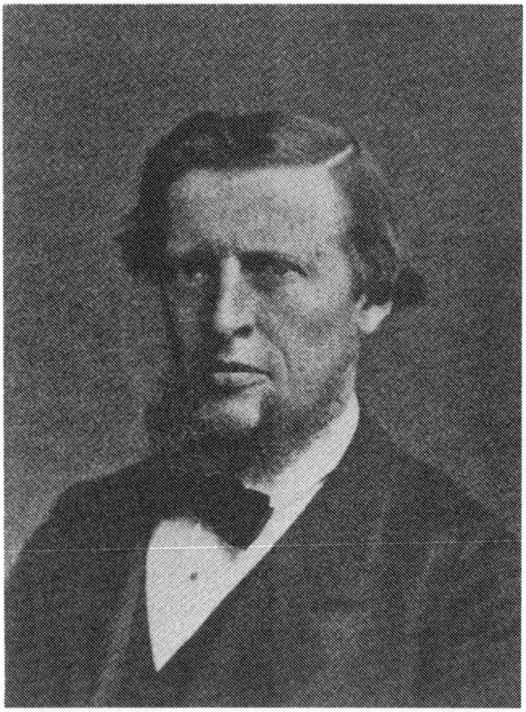

Fig. 1. Dr. Robert Blessig. From: Hirschberg, Vol. III, p. 188.

indeed, eye doctors from all over the western world, including America, Britain, and France trained in Germany. Thomas Shastid discussed some of the progress made in ophthalmology of this time [10]. Hermann von Helmholtz of Königsberg in 1851 published an essay describing his ophthalmoscope. Von Graefe in 1855 used the instrument to describe retinal changes in glaucoma, and in 1856 to assist in performing an iridectomy. Rudolf Virchow studied ocular pathology. In Vienna, Heinrich Kuchler developed visual acuity tests in 1843, modified by Jaeger in 1854, Stellwag von Carion in 1855, and Snellen of Utrecht. All of these advances would find their way into the minds and black bags of expatriate eye doctors and be transplanted to the fertile ground of Russia.

A review of Soviet and American sources reveals that two major factors shaped the course of Russian ophthalmology. The first was widespread eye disease, for which the vast, largely rural Russian Empire had few treatments and fewer public health resources. The second was the respect Russian doctors had for technology, scholarship, and research. Soviet historians particularly show that the doctors who developed ophthalmology in Russia

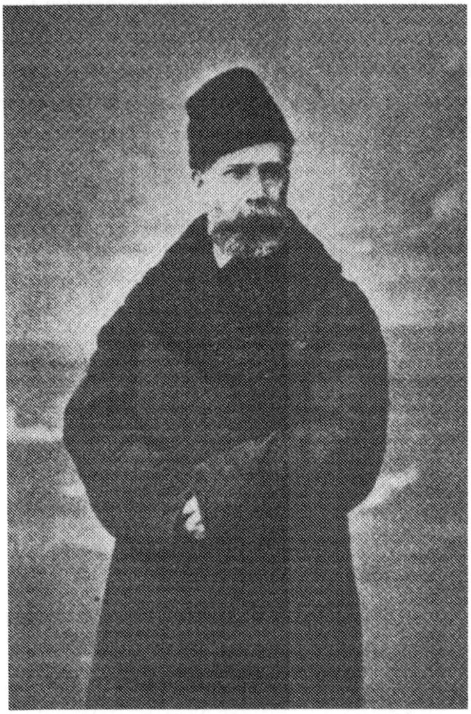

Fig. 2. Dr. S.N. Lozhechnikov. From: Hirschberg, Vol. III, p. 224.

were men of great stature in both academic and public capacities. They trained in Western traditions and worked during times of social change. Their scientific acumen, commitment to the ocular health of the nation, and faith in the medical profession as a means of improving society guided their work. Since their convictions and efforts fitted the principles and programs of the Bolsheviks, Russian ophthalmologists maintained an uninterrupted tradition of training, research, and patient care. Given the support of the new government in 1917, ophthalmology steadily grew in the USSR.

As Nancy Frieden elucidates in her book, Russian medicine before the Nineteenth century was unevenly distributed between gentry and peasantry, and was based on tradition more than science. Medical care was largely imported for the aristocracy, absent from the peasantry. In 1706, Peter I took a first step to provide native Russian medicine by establishing the Military Hospital and Surgical School in Moscow. Consistent with his passion for Western institutions, Peter invited Nicholas Bidloo of Leiden University to direct the school in 1707. This surgeon held the position until 1753 [11]. His appointment, however, did not simply confirm Peter's tastes;

it typified the development of Russian medicine after Peter, featuring state management of medical resources, the contribution of Western doctors and scholarship, and the importance of military medicine. The state built additional military hospitals with corresponding medical academies in St. Petersburg in 1710 and 1733, and in Kronstadt in 1730.

Native medical services and personnel expanded slowly in Russia. The Table of ranks, established in 1722, codified the social standing of physicians and, more importantly, provided a means for their advancement. Under this scheme and its modifications, physicians were able to attain a rank of "minor nobility" [12]. While pay and privileges of doctors did not compare to those of born nobility, physicians could pursue this path which most civil servants could not, and thus achieve nominal recognition for the hazards and sacrifices of medical practice in those days. The menace of the cholera epidemics in 1828–1832 led to two more official actions: an increase in positions in medical academies, and the opening of the ranks to talented students regardless of social standing [13].

During this expansion, the government instituted a policy which affected ophthalmology. The state had controlled production of doctors through its ministries of health, education, and the army. Licenses were first issued in 1721. However, in 1838, the government wrote rules which separated patient care from medical research. These new requirements specified that to receive the degree "Doctor of Medicine," a student had to conduct research and defend a dissertation [14]. Thus, a student could spend five years in medical school, complete an internship, and go into practice (the route of the community care eye doctor), or complete medical school, perform research, defend a dissertation, and go into academia (the route of the institutional ophthalmologist).

Further epidemics of cholera in 1848, and the catastrophic Crimean War of 1853–1856 again drained the meager health resources of the nation. Both crises also influenced the world view and works of Russia's eminent advocate of public health, Nicholas Pirogov. Not only a skillful and influential architect of public policy of his day, Pirogov was also an esteemed scientist and, happily for the specialty, an eye surgeon.

The state carefully controlled medicine in Russia. The government employed most doctors by the last half of the Nineteenth Century. In 1862, Alexander II approved a plan composed by the Committee of Ministers and the Reform Commission to create a system of coordinated, locally-autonomous human service agencies, the *zemstvo*. While the indigenous gentry managed much of the work of the *zemstvo* – schools, orphanages, hospitals, and other institutions – physicians did not answer to it. Doctors kept their independence in part because of a decision by the Ministry of Internal

Affairs (whose ranks included Pirogov) to reserve some authority for the physicians, and in part by the effectiveness of their growing ranks. Both unofficially by weight of numbers and formally through medical societies, doctors pressed for the right to exercise control over their work [15]. In 1867, the *zemstvo* inherited the staff established by the Ministry of State Domains of the 1830's, a cadre of some 350 doctors, 5500 paramedics, 269 clinics, and 1200 rural pharmacies [16]. The work they had initiated expanded, primarily to manage problems such as poor sanitation, cholera, diphtheria, tuberculosis, and infant mortality.

Frieden's discussion reveals three characteristics of Russian medicine which contributed to the growth of Russian ophthalmology. First, the close relationship between doctor and state was essential. This relationship, established under Peter I, provided for the recruitment, education, support, and employment of doctors; it also separated academicians and practitioners. The rise of academia, together with the creation of the *zemstvo*, in part accounted for the rift between research ophthalmologist and community eye doctor. A second factor was the influence of foreign (particularly German) education, research, scholarship, and technology. Also formalized in the days of Peter I, this bond with the West provided training for Russian ophthalmologists, either directly in German institutes or indirectly by German protégés in Russia. Finally, the medical needs of the population shaped the course of ophthalmology.

Soviet articles and Hirschberg discuss early ophthalmologic progress [17]. Dorpat (now Tartu) University in Estonia, under Russian jurisdiction, began training German students in 1628 to be teachers and professors in Russian universities. Its faculties included medical and surgical departments. Within the department of surgery, doctors began specializing in eye operations in 1802. The first doctor formally seated as a professor of ophthalmology was M.E. Kautsman, who served from 1805–1810. He was followed by I.L. Jochman, 1811–1814; Johan Christian Moier, 1814–1836; and Professor Nicholas Pirogov, 1836–1841. A chair in ophthalmology was created apart from the surgery department in 1843 under the guidance of G. Adelman, who taught at Dorpat from 1841–1871 [18]. German technology came quickly in this period. A student of Helmholtz, G. Ettingen brought the ophthalmoscope to Estonia in 1855. At the university he organized eye care from 1856–1859, and in 1867, he and fellow professor George Fonn (1855–1867 at Dorpat) oversaw the creation of a separate department of ophthalmology.

Riga, in the Baltic state of Latvia, also enjoyed German influence, although eye care was dispensed in the community more than in universities. The first clinic opened in 1857 under C. Waldehauer. He and his successors

J. Stavenhagen (1870) and L. Mandelshtam (1874), kept it a private institution, although they cooperated with the Riga City Hospital [19]. The ophthalmologists in the clinic were German, German-trained, or educated in the German tradition. A good example of the latter is Karl Dalfeld, a Latvian from Riga who was educated abroad and received his doctorate from Dorpat in 1885 after defense of a dissertation on trachoma. He returned to Riga in 1887 to practice ophthalmology. He studied the value of X-rays in locating foreign bodies from 1896–1897 [20]. The distinction of developing radiology for Latvia, however, belongs to Nicholas Port, a Riga-educated chemist who experimented with X-rays in 1897, following Roentgen's lead. Port conducted his work at Riga City Hospital [21].

The Baltic states' longstanding ties with the West provided one pathway for the entry of German scholarship into the Russian empire. Dorpat produced ophthalmologists who moved to St. Petersburg, Moscow, and Kiev to perform research and practice medicine. Such graduates included Pirogov, Blessig, Ettingen, Mandelshtam, and others. They not only trained in the Western traditions of Estonia, but many also pursued postgraduate study in Germany. As well, Dorpat and Riga provide a glimpse of early research and technology in Russian ophthalmology. The gap between research and the care of peoples' eyes, however, was wider in Russia.

The earliest eye specialists in northern Russia worked at the Medical-Surgical Academy of St. Petersburg. The institution was established in 1798. A modest facility of three rooms, it included a ward with twelve beds, a closet for storage of instruments, and a lecture hall which also served as an operating room. One of its founders, Professor I.F. Bush (1771–1843), practiced general and ocular surgery. Not until 1805, however, when Peter Frank (1745–1821) became president of the Academy, did a position for an ophthalmologist open. Frank's initiative also increased the number of departments in the Academy from seven to fourteen, and improved the facilities. Alexander I approved this expansion in 1806; in 1818, he also authorized a chair in ophthalmology at the Academy, held by Professor I.E. Grubi (1755–1834). Grubi succeeded in acquiring instruments for his specialty from the department of surgery, and worked with the optician Reichenbach in 1830 to develop special tools for diagnosis. In 1806, the St. Petersburg Eye Infirmary was founded. One of its early leaders was William F. Froebelius (1812–1886), a St. Petersburg native who graduated from Dorpat University and, in 1842, headed the institution (see Fig. 3). He performed the earliest iridectomy in Russia (1857) and devised improvements to the ophthalmoscope [22]. After Froebelius, Robert Blessig (1830)–1878) directed the hospital. Born in Petersburg, Blessig graduated from Dorpat in 1855. He undertook postgraduate eye training in Germany under

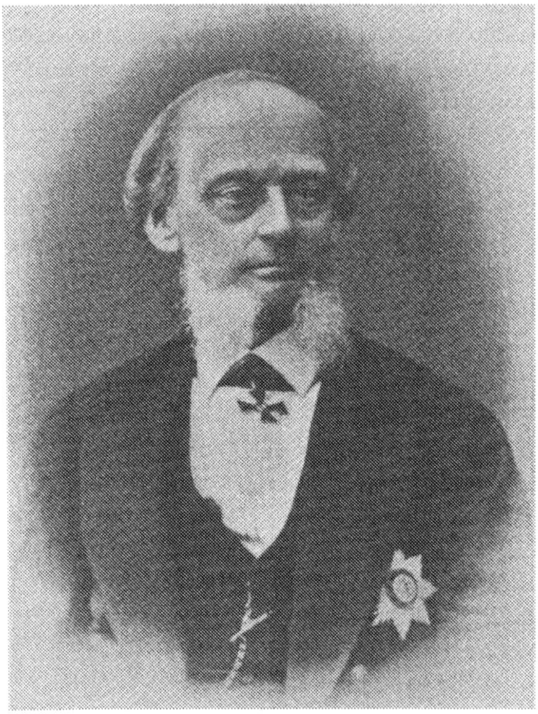

Fig. 3. Dr. Wilhelm Froebelius. From: Hirschberg, Vol. III, p. 195.

Virchow, Arlt and Graefe. He returned to Petersburg, where, in 1863, he became chief physician of the eye infirmary. In 1855, he described peripheral cystoid degeneration of the retina, a pathological entity which today bears his name [23]. In 1878, Blessig acquired typhus from a patient during surgery, and died later that year.

Ophthalmology concerned other institutions in Petersburg. Ivan Kabat, head of the eye clinic of the Petersburg Military Academy from 1812–1844, promoted eye care and science in the army and navy. In 1857, he attended the first International Congress of Ophthalmology, returning to Russia with the first ophthalmoscope in Petersburg (a year after Ettingen brought one to Dorpat). Because of his Western connections, Kabat had access to Graefe's manuscript on iridectomy, which he translated and published in *Voenno-meditsinskij zhurnal* (Military Medicine Journal) in 1858. Subsequently he performed the operation on a glaucoma patient, Peter Chesnokov, who had suffered from the disease since 1852 [24]. An outstanding heir of Kabat was Eduard Junge (1832–1898), a Latvian from Riga who graduated from Moscow State University and subsequently studied under

Virchow, Helmholtz, Müller, and Graefe. He returned in 1859 as chairman of the Moscow department of ophthalmology, and saw to it that his graduates practiced in every military district in the empire [25]. Among his pupils were Vladimir Ivanovich Dobrovolskij, A.V. Chodin, and Reich. Junge used his influence to produce a chair in ophthalmology in all university departments of surgery. In addition to his clinical and educational work, he conducted research on the disease retinitis pigmentosa. His tenure ended in 1882, and his student V.I. Dobrovolskij (1838–1904) followed him in 1883. Dobrovolskij is best known for his research in amblyopia, astigmatism, myopia, and physiology of the retina. One of his 1886 graduates, L.G. Belliarminov (1859–1930) succeeded him to the chair of the department.

More conspicuously than in Dorpat or Riga, the ties between German ophthalmologist-researchers and Russian aspirants were found in Petersburg. Petersburg had an important part in educating the Russian doctors who would specialize in eyes and eventually teach other Russians. The oculists of Petersburg at this time tended to serve two roles; while they were trained in science and eager to pursue it, their responsibilities for eye care for specialized urban populations (soldiers and nobility) interfered with that calling. Also, public health facilities for eyes began in Petersburg, from a mere twelve beds in 1798, to an empire-wide network of military and university clinics by the turn of the century.

Moscow was less illustrious in early Russian ophthalmology than Petersburg or Dorpat. Three facilities served ocular needs there in the Nineteenth Century. The oldest was the Moscow Eye Infirmary, founded in 1826 by Basse and directed by him for 34 years [26]. His successor, S.N. Lozhechnikov was a naturalized citizen from Germany. In 1892, the New Moscow City Eye Clinic opened. This institution had 34 beds, a clinic, and an ambulance. Alexander Nicholaevich Maklakov (1832–1959) (see Fig. 4), ophthalmologist, member of the Duma, and painter, led the clinic [27]. Contemporary ophthalmologists knew Maklakov for his invention, the applanation tonometer. Introduced in 1884 in *Meditsinskoe obozrenie* (Medical Review), Maklakov's instrument offered greater accuracy in gauging intraocular pressure by measuring from the sclera rather than the cornea. While the Schiotz tonometer superseded Maklakov's invention in 1905, it was a much-celebrated device in its day. Equipped with his tonometer, Maklakov invited S.S. Golovin to join him in 1892, and jointly they studied the effects of drugs (atropine, pilocarpine, eserine, and cocaine) on intraocular pressure. This work led to Golovin's dissertation "Ophthalmotonometric Research" in 1895 [28]. Maklakov died in 1895, and the clinic passed to A.A. Kruikov (1849–1908), who studied color vision, spherical aberration, and muscle strength. Kruikov wrote a major textbook on eye

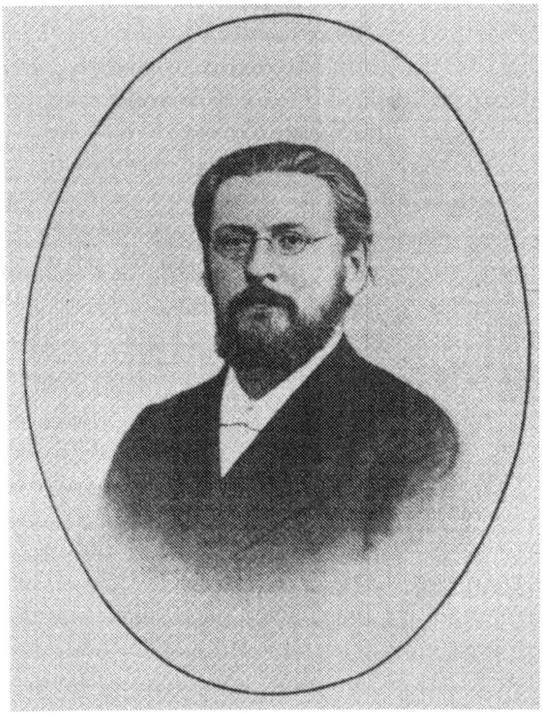

Fig. 4. Prof. A.N. Malakov. From: Hirschberg, Vol. III, p. 217.

disease, one of the first ophthalmologic texts printed in Russian [29]. Kruikov also founded the Moscow Society of Eye Doctors in 1857 [30].

The third eye clinic in Moscow, the Municipal Eye Hospital, was created as the result of a gift by Mrs. R. Alekseev in 1900. A. Natikson (1862–1909) initially directed this 47-bed facility, but anti-Semitism hampered his management [31]. The Helmholtz Institute eventually incorporated much of the Alekseev Hospital.

Moscovite ophthalmologist Gustav Braun (1827–1897) made another contribution. A graduate of Moscow State University, postdoctoral student of Graefe and Donders, and professor of ophthalmology at Moscow State University for 33 years, Braun wrote the first textbook of ophthalmology in Russian in 1859 [32]. His research interests included glaucoma and cataracts.

In central Russia, Moscow oculists practiced ophthalmology different from that of the north. While eye doctors in St. Petersburg and Dorpat participated in research, teaching, and patient care, Muscovites favored direct delivery of eye services. Doctors in both northern and central Russia, however, focused their work on limited populations in cities. In southern

Russia (Kiev, Odessa, and Kharkov), oculists practiced a wide array of research, patient treatment, and rural care.

One early leading eye doctor in Kiev was Christian von Hubennet (1822–1873). A veteran surgeon of the Crimean War and associate of Pirogov, he was naturalized as a citizen after he emigrated from Germany. He served as professor of ophthalmology and surgery from 1851 to 1869 at Kiev University. He is credited with bringing the first ophthalmoscope and artificial eyes to Russia in 1852 [33]. His contemporary, Vladimir Karavaev (1811–1893), directed the eye clinic which was associated with the department of surgery at the University. Under his influence, the departments separated in 1869 [34], and he became director of the new eye division. An able administrator and surgeon, Karavaev practiced and taught modern cataract extraction in preference to the outdated "couching" technique [35]. Andrei Ivanov followed him (1836–1880). A graduate of Moscow State University (1859) and student of Heinrich Müller of Germany, Ivanov came to Kiev in 1869 to conduct research on pathology of the retina and optic nerve. He shared credit with Robert Blessig for the study of retinal pathology [36]. Because he suffered progressive tuberculosis, he took academic leave in 1876. He died in Germany. His temporary replacement, Emanuel Mandelshtam (1839–1912) practided ophthalmology in Kiev from 1875–1880. Born to a Jewish merchant family in Kovro, Mandelshtam studied medicine at Dorpat and defended his dissertation in St. Petersburg in 1868. When Ivanov died, the faculty elected Mandelshtam to the chairmanship of the department, but eventually denied him the position because he was Jewish [37]. A.V. Chodin (1847–1905), a student of Junge's in Petersburg, took over. As a physiologist, Chodin conducted research on color vision. In addition to his studies, Chodin founded one of the leading journals of ophthalmology in Russia, *Vestnik oftalmologii* (Annals of Ophthalmology), in 1884. He retired in 1902.

Heinrich Stieda came to Odessa in 1867 to practice eye surgery [38]. In 1875 he oversaw the creation of a 90-bed eye infirmary. Not until 1903, however, with the foundation of the new Russian University and its department of ophthalmology did the specialty excel in Odessa. The department grew under the direction of Professor Sergei Semjonovich Golovin [39]. Another important scholar followed him in 1911, Vladimir Petrovich Filatov. He directed this department and the Odessa Medical Institute until 1936. This institution produced the Ukrainian Research Institute of Eye Diseases in 1939, which Filatov led until his death in 1956 [40].

Italian surgeon T.L. Vanzetti (1809–1888) came to Odessa in 1835 as the personal physician of Count M.S. Vorontsov. Academia called him away from Odessa in 1838, however; he joined the medical faculty of Kharkov

[41]. From then until 1853, he read his lectures in Latin and practiced at the University. The Crimean War forced Vanzetti to return to Italy; thus, he did not participate in the inauguration of the new eye department at Kharkov in 1868. Leonard L. Girshman (1839–1921), a German, holds the distinction of being its first chairman. He graduated from Kharkov University in 1860. Following receipt of his diploma, he studied in Germany with Graefe, Virchow, and Helmholtz. Girshman defended his dissertation "Materials for the Physiology of Color Vision" in 1868. The new department received ten beds from the department of surgery [42]. Its facilities expanded in 1880 when the Kharkov *zemstvo* organized a special hospital for the University.

Women in southern Russia in the Nineteenth Century trained as doctors and eye specialists in large numbers. An example was Olga Arkadeovna Mashkotseva (1851–1933) [43]. A student of Dobrovolskij's in Petersburg and 1878 graduate of the Nicholas Army Hospital, she practiced in Simeropol from 1887 to 1933. Active in the new eye societies, she made many presentations of case histories at regional and national meetings. She was an "eye doctor," however, who pursued primary care rather than research. Evgenija Elizarovna Dickenskaja also studied in Petersburg. She graduated in 1883 and, in 1888, went to Kherson. She joined the "flying squads," a unit of doctors and nurses which travelled through underserved areas to treat disease. Dickenskaja published a paper in 1897, "Summary of the Activities of the Flying Squad of Oculists in the Zakaspijskaja Region in 1896" [44]. Dickenskaja, Mashkotseva, and most of the women oculists of their time, completed the five-year medical course and perhaps a year of semi-specialized internship, then went into practice. Their part in providing service expanded in the Soviet era.

The example of the Ukraine demonstrates several important features of Russian ophthalmology. Here, too, Germany contributed to eye science, as many leading figures were immigrant or ethnic Germans. Research and technology enjoyed special favor. The Ukraine was first in Russia to gain the ophthalmoscope; modern procedures and operations were practiced and taught in the Ukraine. Also, numerous departments in universities and some of the first eye institutes were founded in the Ukraine; academicians there conducted important research.

The value placed on research and the clinical needs of the country propelled ophthalmology in Russia. Also, many leaders in the development of public health services in Russia were ophthalmologists as well. Outstanding among these are Nicholas Pirogov, Sergei Golovin, Leonid Belliarminov, and Vladimir Filatov.

Nicholas Ivanovich Pirogov is better remembered as an "eye surgeon" than as an ophthalmologist. He took his training at Dorpat on the invitation of the Dutch ophthalmologist Johann Christian Moier, but Pirogov's background included medicine, surgery, anatomy and pathology. Indeed, in his memoirs, Pirogov devoted far more attention to the surgery he practiced for antiseptic amputation on the battlefields of the Crimea than he did to the cataract extractions with which he is credited [45]. Born in 1810, Pirogov went to Moscow State University in 1824. In 1827 he began his study of medicine at the University's Professor Institute. He followed this program with advanced work and research at Dorpat. He defended his dissertation on arterial trunks and the aorta in 1833, then pursued postgraduate education in Berlin and Göttingen for two years. In 1836 Pirogov returned to the department of surgery in Dorpat at Moier's request, accepting a position he kept until 1841 [46]. He published many works during this period, including studies on surgery, anatomy, and pathology. One piece which he considered particularly important was a paper on anesthesia in animals, in which ether was passed by rectum to induce surgical sleep. In 1847, V.V. Pelikan requested that Pirogov leave academia for public service in the Department of Military Medicine. Pirogov worked for the Department in the Caucasus. Here, war exerted a powerful influence on Pirogov, and twice it took him from administration and forced him into stressful clinical settings. War in the East (1851–1852) and the Crimean War (1853–1856) taught Pirogov principles of combat surgery of all kinds, and provided him a basis for developing a system of battlefield management for the wounded. He published his conclusions in 1863. In the years following the wars, Pirogov served in various divisions of the government, including the Ministry of Education, the Ministry of Internal Affairs, the Military Medicine Department, and others. His public career ended in 1866, when he was forced to resign because of his liberal political stands [47]. He died in 1881.

While Pirogov's contribution to the science and practice of ophthalmology can only be evaluated in the broader context of his work in anatomy and surgery, his contribution to public health and well-being was substantial. A liberal in times of reform, he eloquently advocated policies which would increase the quantity and accessibility of medical care to the Russians. His memoirs are riddled with criticism of the disservice that bureaucracy did to the physicians in the field. He also devoted much thought to public education at all levels, including health issues and general literacy [48]. Pirogov had great faith in the value of education in transforming Russia, but much frustration at the state's sluggish pace of social reform. Revered by his colleagues, Pirogov's name was given to the national organization of physicians founded in 1883, two years after his death.

One of those contemporaries who shared Pirogov's dedication to education, public health, and national enlightenment was Sergei Semjonovich

Golovin. Unlike Pirogov, Golovin devoted his professional life to ophthalmology. He began his career in 1890 at Moscow's Kutajskaja Hospital. He produced a public education brochure in 1892, "Save Your Eyes," and also began his study with Maklakov on the effects of various drugs on intraocular pressure. This study culminated in his 1895 dissertation, "Ophthalmotonometric Research." Golovin entered private practice that year, but left it in 1903 to assume the chair at the eye clinic at New Russian University of Odessa. His research in the University was substantial. Publications included "Tumors of the Optic Nerve and Their Surgical Treatment" (1904), "Incidence of the Application of Roentgenography in Cases of a Foreign Body in the Eye" (1905), "On Cysts of the Ethmoid Labyrinth" (1907), and "Continuous Exenteration of the Orbits and Their Neighboring Cavities" (1907) [49].

Under Golovin's stewardship, the department saw the production of fifty scientific studies and the defense of four dissertations, including V.P. Filatov's "The Study of Cellular Toxins in Ophthalmology" in 1908 [50]. In 1911, Golovin returned to Moscow, where he worked at the University-affiliated City Eye Hospital until 1918. He left to assume a professorship at the First Medical Institute of Moscow (1919–1925). He concluded his academic career at Moscow State University, where he served in the eye clinic, and at New Eketerinskaja Hospital from 1925 to 1930. He died from a heart condition which had troubled him for thirteen years [51].

While Golovin is remembered for his extensive research, refinements of surgery (particularly exenteration and enucleation), and cadre of trainees (including Verbitskij, Judin, Dmitriev, and Filatov), perhaps the peak of his career was an address which he delivered at the inauguration of the New Russian University in Odessa. Not just an accomplishment for Golovin, the address heralded the transformation of ophthalmologic care in Russia.

Read on September 25, 1903, the speech attempted "to show you the measure of the evil to which ophthalmology calls us to do battle" [52]. Golovin based his lecture on several years of epidemiologic and sociologic research drawn from the military, the census, the outlying eye clinics, and his experience. After the speech, Golovin continued his research and published it in 1910. In his report, "On Blindness in Russia," Golovin outlined the causes of blindness in the nation and called for action to eradicate them. An important work which ophthalmologists would cite until the 1960's, it deserves review.

Golovin began by describing previous efforts to count the blind in Russia. The earliest took place in 1855 in the Dorpat principality under the direction of S. von Himmelstern. Studies were also made in the military; the journal *Skrebitskij* reported in 1879 and 1880 that of 444 blind soldiers studied, five percent lost their vision due to battle, the remainder due to infection [53]. In 1881, the Trusteeship of Empress Maria Aleksandrovna for the Blind made an attempt to count the sightless. This institution investigated districts such as Kiev and Kazan, and in 1886 performed the first complete census of the blind for European Russia. Important scholars in this effort included Dobrovolskij and Belliarminov. Their definition of blindness for this study involved "one suffering from irreversible weakening of the vision in both eyes which does not allow him to count fingers beyond one-third of a meter" [54].

Golovin presented data from the 1886 study and the general census of 1897. Golovin found that 20/10 000 people were blind; the lowest density was in Warsaw (2–3/10 000) and the highest was in Kazan (95/10 000). This tally compared poorly to that of the average incidence of blindness in the West, which was 9.4/10 000 (4.5/10 000 in Holland, 8.1/10 000 in Germany, 8.8/10 000 in England, and 9.8/10 000 in America) [55].

Golovin investigated climate, lifestyle, geography, industrial exposure, alcohol use, and other factors as they related to blindness. He found, however, that nationality and level of public sanitation were crucial. The non-European, rural Votjakov had an incidence of 83/10 000; the Tatar 51/10 000. Russians were 19/10 000 blind; Germans only 7/10 000. Class also played a role. Peasants comprised 86 percent of the sightless, bourgeoisie 5.5 percent, soldiers 3.8 percent, and landowners and clergy less than one percent. Blindness tended to a polar distribution, with large groups under five years of age and over 65 years. Of the 247 000 blind estimated in 1897, Golovin counted 71 000 blind from birth, 176 000 acquired [56].

To determine the causes of blindness in the Empire, Golovin drew on four study groups. The first consisted of patients recorded by the Trusteeship of Empress Marie Aleksandrovna, 1893–1906. The next group came from similar institutions, 1897–1906. Private patients were studied, 1878–1906. Finally, Golovin followed a small group of patients specifically for the project in 1887–1899. The etiologies of blindness as elucidated by these 65 724 cases were trachoma (21.4 percent), glaucoma (19.2 percent), diseases of the cornea (13.5 percent), smallpox (12.1 percent), and others (suppuration of the newborn, disease of the optic nerve and central nervous system, vascular disease, syphilis, injury, and congenital) [57]. These leading causes of blindness compared poorly to those in Europe. In Germany, trachoma accounted for only 9.4 percent of blindness, glaucoma 8.9 percent, corneal disease 8.0 percent, and smallpox 2.2 percent. In France, the statistics were trachoma 1.9 percent, glaucoma 19 percent, corneal disease 8 percent, and smallpox 1.1 percent. In short, infectious trachoma and smallpox were not leading causes of blindness in the West [58].

Golovin noted that dangers of city life threatened the vision of the urbanite (industrial risk, pollution, trauma, syphilis, and so on), while inaccessibility of eye care menaced the peasant's vision. The lower classes suffered from eye disease because of hard and dangerous work, crowded living, poor sanitation, and inadequate education. Often the uneducated would attempt to treat eye ailments with saliva, milk, animal blood, or earthworms. The doctor observed, "It is demonstrated by the available statistics that the blind in the vast majority of cases are underprivileged people" [59].

Golovin expressed three concerns about ocular morbidity: personal hardship, economic drain, and inadequate personnel for the army. He believed blindness to be a "great evil" in Russia, and proposed three general reforms to contain it.

The first was education. Data and experience suggested to Golovin that blindness was an affliction of the illiterate. Thus, he recommended general education and propagation of public health information. Second, Golovin called for improved sanitation in all factories, schools, towns, and cities. Adequate hygiene had to be provided if infectious diseases were to be controlled. Finally, Golovin recommended an increase in the number of oculists, hospitals, beds, clinics, and institutes. He stressed the importance of accessibility to these resources. Golovin called on the eye specialty societies (the first of which in the Ukraine was founded in 1893) and the universities to provide thorough ophthalmologic education to medical students, including therapy for the most menacing diseases. He noted that in 1870, German medical professors had gathered in Stuttgart to outline a rigorous education for ophthalmologists. Golovin believed a similar meeting should be held in Russia.

Golovin finished his report with details about management of specific causes of blindness: congenital, blennorrhea neonatorum, trachoma, corneal disease, glaucoma, vascular disease, injury, syphilis, and smallpox. He concluded by forcefully restating this three tenets: the evil of blindness in Russia was great; battle with the evil was possible and could be successful; and Russia was woefully ill-equipped to do battle [60].

Golovin's attitude epitomized Russian medicine. The statistics and observations reported the state of health care, sanitation, and services in Russia; but, as well, the contents and tone revealed how doctors perceived their role in the nation. The moral indignation that Golovin felt about his country's medical and social shortcomings is compelling. He, and many of his contemporaries, saw medicine as not just the technical care for disease, but as a means of transforming Russian society. It was not enough for the Golovins and Pirogovs of the country to call for more doctors and better facilities; they demanded as well national enlightenment, and called for state-supported education and protection of the underprivileged to raise the dawn over the darkness of the recent feudal past.

Leonid Georgievich Belliarminov (1859–1930) exemplified the character and work of the socially-aware physician of the day. While not as publicly visible as Pirogov or Golovin, Belliarminov nevertheless made substantial contributions. Born in Saratovskij region, he studied medicine at the Medical-Surgical Academy in St. Petersburg, graduating in 1883 with honors [61]. The prevalence of ocular disease in his home province impressed him and stimulated his interest in specializing in eyes. He undertook research in physiology with I.P. Tarkhanov for three years. This work led to his dissertation in 1886, "The Experience of the Application of the Graphic Method to the Study of the Movement of the Pupil and Intraocular Pressure." Concomitantly he published, "On the Suitability and Accuracy of the Existing Eye Charts for the Determination of Visual Acuity." Belliarminov subsequently spent two years (1886–1888) studying with Helmholtz and Virchow in Germany, and with Becker, Leber, and Ginsberg in Russia. [62]. During this period he worked on the epidemiologic studies of blindness that were so important to Golovin's work. In 1888 Belliarminov returned to the St. Peterburg Medical-Surgical Academy, where he became a professor of ophthalmology and, from 1893–1923, director of the department. He collaborated with A.I. Mertsov during this tenure to produce the three-volume *Eye Diseases* [63].

In 1892 Belliarminov conceived a plan to send "flying squads" into the country to tend to the ocular needs of the peasants [64]. These squads consisted of two-to-three ophthalmologists, one-to-two assistants, and one or two nurses. They would treat a community or region for two-to-three months and then move to another. In 1893, the *zemstvo* organized seven "flying squads" and rotated them through the country [65]. While too few in number, the squads did remarkable work. When World War I came, the army used this organization, under Belliarminov's direction, to manage the eye injuries and diseases of the troops. Three squads were created for this purpose [66].

In addition to his scholarship and public works, Belliarminov dedicated himself to teaching. His students produced many papers and dissertations; eleven later became professors and led departments throughout the nation. Outstanding examples were N.I. Androgskij and Ja. V. Zelenkovskij in Petersburg; A.S. Chemolosov in Smolensk; S.V. Ochapovskij in Krasnodar; I.I. Kazas in Ekaterinoslav/Dnepropetrovsk; and A.G. Trutin in Baku.

The fourth figure of Russian ophthalmology saw the turn of the century and the Revolution, and was active well into the Soviet era. Vladimir

Petrovich Filatov was born in 1875 in Mikhajlovsk, a town in the Penzenskij region, the son of a *zemstvo* doctor [67]. Filatov spent his formative years in the country, where he saw the suffering that eye disease brought to his father's practice. Filatov studied medicine at Odessa, completing his training in 1908 under Golovin with his dissertation "The Study of Cellular Toxins in Ophthalmology" [68]. He continued his career there, primarily in research and surgery. Filatov's career reflected the changes brought by the Revolution: the increased respect for research, and the expansion of the rolls of eye doctors who practiced the specialty in the field, enabling academicians to work more in the laboratory. Filatov worked there until his death in 1956.

The men and women who studied and treated eyes in Russia in this period addressed many challenges which the Soviet Union would inherit as the eye doctors had already defined them. The leading issue, as eloquently delineated by Golovin, was the deplorable medical-social milieu which permitted so much eye disease. The problems of trachoma, glaucoma, smallpox, tuberculosis, and other illnesses posed formidable barriers to the progress of public health. The concern of inadequate personnel and facilities was paramount. In 1917 there were some 300 ophthalmologists and 2000 beds for eye patients in Russia [69]. There were eleven university-based departments of ophthalmology. Academicians had excellent training, but the community care eye doctors generally had to learn as they practiced. Delivery of services was awkward and uneven. While urban populations had modest access to eye specialists, the rural folk depended on the "flying squads." Follow-up services and continuity of care were also lacking. For example, the therapy for trachoma required serial treatments of rubbing the conjunctiva and affected sclera with a copper sulfate pencil, or alternatively dousing the eye with silver nitrate. These specialized procedures demanded skill and training to perform – that is, they required a doctor to be present for the whole treatment regimen [70]. Obviously, a "flying squad" which would depart in a matter of weeks or months could not provide long-term care. Military medicine also continued to be a concern; Pirogov, Hubennet, Belliarminov, Filatov, and scores of other ophthalmologists practiced their specialty in the armed forces. A distinguished military ophthalmologist, Joseph Talko, documented the crisis in the army in 1893, showing that 871 000 soldiers and 36 000 officers suffered from treatable eye disease, mainly catarrhal conjunctivitis (48.8 percent) and trachoma conjunctivitis (36.5 percent) [71]. This situation led to Golovin's concern in his report "On Blindness in Russia" about the consequences of ocular disability to national security.

By the end of the Nineteenth Century, professionalization became an issue. While ophthalmology came into its own in the 1840's by the creation of eye departments, eye doctors did not associate as specialists until later. Some early organizations appeared in St. Petersburg: The Russian Ophthalmologic Society in 1885, the German Ophthalmologic Society in 1886. Interestingly, the latter was the larger group [72]. Ophthalmology was recognized as a routine part of medical practice by 1876; the state took measures that year to increase enrollments in medical schools, offering scholarships, stipends, a black bag with instruments, and a personal ophthalmoscope to all students [73]. The split between community eye care doctors and academicians became wider as the century progressed; however, the two groups' interests complemented each other. And because each group appealed to a specific need and value which the Soviets embraced, both grew in the Twentieth Century.

During the Revolution, some ophthalmologists were bona fide radicals. V.M. Krutovskij (1856–1945) was sent to Siberia for revolutionary activities; he established his practice there, settling in Krasnojarsk and founding a doctors' society in 1886 [74]. K.A. Belilovskij (1859–1938) was born in Poljashchin, graduated from medical school in 1883, and in 1894 became a professor of medicine and surgery in St. Petersburg. In 1905 he was arrested for subversive activity (including his poetry and publications) and exiled to Olonetskaja principality. Following the Revolution, he joined the Commissary of Foreign Affairs [75]. I.I. Ginsberg (1869–1929) studied medicine in Kiev, but was expelled for student agitation. He moved to Moscow, whence he graduated in 1887, a student of Maklakov and Lozhechnikov. He practiced ophthalmology in the Vorzhenskaya Hospital 1889–1905, but was imprisoned for eight years on charges of subversion. Following his release, he was threatened with internal exile, which compelled him to leave the country for three years. Ginsberg spent his time with Fuchs in Vienna and Hirschberg in Berlin. Following the 1917 Revolution, he returned to Kiev, where he studied radiology of the eye [76]. S.M. Sanovich (1878–1932) was arrested in 1899 for revolutionary activity. He went on to chair the All-Ukrainian Institute in Memory of Girshman, as well as to direct the eye clinic in Kharkov and the Advanced Training Institute for Ophthalmologists [77]. A.I. Pokrovskij (1880–1958) was expelled from Moscow State University and imprisoned in Taganskij for his political leanings. During the Revolution, he joined the Soviet of Workers and Soldiers Deputies of the Fergan region and led local medical societies. In 1951, he became a member of the Supreme Soviet of the Russian Soviet Federated Socialist Republic [78].

These cases are the extremes; by-and-large, Russian ophthalmologists and doctors in general were not known for their frankly subversive or revolutionary activities. However, many were revolutionary in a social, if not political, sense; that is, they criticized the inertia of the state and of institutions which perpetuated medieval relationships between gentry and masses. These doctors included men of great stature, including Pirogov, Golovin, Belliarminov, Maklakov, and others. They were revolutionary in a scientific sense, as well, because they adopted technology and research as their tools in the 1850's, long before the Bolsheviks came to support those endeavors.

The Soviet commitment to science can be traced from the earliest days of the USSR. In a speech delivered 26 May, 1918, shortly after his rise to power, Lenin related the arrival of socialism to the liberation of the sciences. He elaborated in an address on 1 March 1920, in which he proposed that socialism would provide a context in which workers and scientists could forge freedom from disease [79]. His theories materialized in August 1918 when Lenin created the Peoples Committee of Public Health from the Soviet Academy of Medical Scientists. L.A. Tarasevich led this committee.

As Mark Field points out, the Soviets demanded the disappearance of distinction between theory and practice in their research, and they required the planning of scientific activity on a national basis. They equated pure science with bourgeois parasitism; thus, research had to have tangible clinical benefits [80]. Fortunately, ophthalmologic research had practiced this principle for years. In 1918 the Peoples Committee of Public Health established a division on eye diseases. The Committee appointed Ja. F. Globa director in 1920, and he planned a national strategy for management of trachoma. The plan included increased clinical practice and increased research [81].

Before the Revolution, research institutes were few. The first was the Bacteriologic Institute of the Kharkov Medical Society, founded in 1887; the Institute of Experimental Medicine in St. Petersburg followed in 1890, where Pavlov worked and developed a theory of visual perception as a conditioned reflex; in 1895 the Moscow Bacteriologic Institute. In all, there were twelve institutes dedicated to scientific research in tsarist Russia; none studied eyes exclusively [82].

The Soviets, embracing a commitment to research and inheriting a legacy of serious public health problems, began promptly to create institutes which would meet the urgent needs of the nation. In 1918, the Institute of Microbiology and Epidemiology in the Struggle against Plague was founded under Saratov [83]. The Institute of Experimental Medicine and Control of Sera and Vaccine followed in 1919, then the Central Smallpox Institute in 1920. Eighteen new research centers for infectious disease were organized from 1917–1920 [84]. The move was advantageous for ophthalmologists; given their concerns with trachoma, smallpox, tuberculosis, and other communicable diseases, they readily staffed appropriate institutes. In 1922 came the Trachoma Institute in Kazan under V.V. Chikovskij [85]. He moved to Leningrad later to direct the Research Institute in Memory of Girshman. Kharkov followed with the Ukrainian Institute in Memory of Girshman in 1930 under I.I. Merkulov. The Moscow City Eye Hospital founded by Mrs. Alekseev's gift moved toward research, and in 1929 was refounded as the Moscow Research Institute in memory of Helmholtz under M.I. Averbakh. Filatov's Ukrainian Institute in Odessa began in 1931 with an antiglaucoma division. V.P. Odintsov, ocular pathologist of the First Moscow Medical Institute, founded the Bashkir Trachoma Institute in Ufa, directed by V.I. Spaskij; another, the Turkmen Trachoma Institute, opened in Ashkhabad in 1932 under K.I. Tsikulenko. The Kazakh Eye Institute started later in Alma-Ata, directed by V.P. Roshchin [86].

In the early days after the Revolution, Soviet Institutes emphasized epidemiology, microbiology, and infectious disease. The first centers dedicated to eyes dealt particularly with trachoma. Appropriately, these institutes were placed in areas of high morbidity, such as the underdeveloped Turkmen, Kazakstan, and rural Ukraine. Urban centers with hospitals for infectious disease, for example Moscow and Kiev, built institutes which pursued academic work in treating disease.

In spite of the effort, the task of controlling eye disease was enormous. A follow-up study based on the 1926 census compared the state of ocular health in the new USSR and that in the old tsarist Russia of Golovin's day. In the Soviet era, blindness had decreased to 234 000 people, from 247 00 in 1897. The leading causes, however, remained trachoma, glaucoma, smallpox, corneal disease, and blennorrhea neonatorum, in that order [87].

Treatments and their delivery increased in the 1920–1930's. Vladimir Filatov had dreamed of corneal transplantation in his student days, and began to practice corneal grafting in 1912 in Odessa [88]. World War I interrupted the work however, and it didn't resume until 1922. Grafting became a common procedure by the 1930's. In another of his projects, Filatov practiced "tissue therapy" in 1933–1938 [89]. He began with human homografts in his corneal surgeries, later attempting animal xenografts. The therapy required isolating a piece of tissue from a source other than the eye and subjecting it to a nonphysiologic challenge – heat, cold, acidity, or other – and grafting it to the field of corneal surgery. In theory, the challenge evoked "biogenic stimulators" in the tissue, which when grafted to the endangered area facilitated regeneration and healing [90]. While Filatov did not elaborate on the mechanism of "tissue therapy," it was considered a serious treatment.

Scientists studied other diseases and their therapies. Reports on trachoma, tuberculosis, and glaucoma persisted in *Vestnik oftalmologii.* In spite of the progress made in treatment and accessibility, these diseases continued to cause blindness. In order to combat them, the government produced institutes and by 1940 had 63 departments of eye disease in universities, 3212 eye specialists, and 13 015 beds for eye patients (compared to no institutes, few departments, 300 doctors, and 2000 beds before 1917) [91]. Regardless, the problems diminished to levels acceptable to the People's Committee on Public Health only in the 1960's. Research into other diseases yield therapies exotic in the Western view: vitamin B1 for glaucoma in 1938, exercises for reduction of intraocular pressure in 1937, injections of fish oil for degenerative disease in 1939 [92]. As well, basic research was carried out and reported assiduously in the areas of pathologic anatomy, anatomic anomalies, chemistry of the lens, strabismus, cataracts, neurology of the eye, and others.

There was substantial political content in ophthalmology in the 1920–1930's as well. In general, the doctors' review of the government was favorable; the Soviet dream of catching up with the West in health and research met with approval among the eye doctors. While it is clear that most ophthalmologists were not politicians, those in influential positions had liberal values and hopes which were acceptable to the Communist government. Thus, the political commentary of *Vestnik oftalmologii* in the 1930's was tolerant. The Party Congresses were reported, articles from Stalin appeared, ophthalmologist "heroes of socialist labor" were extolled.

War brought ocular trauma and surgical complications to the attention of researchers and clinicians [93]. In February of 1941, the Helmholtz Institute in Moscow began work with the army to develop a protocol for management of injuries to the eye. It was functional by 1942, and involved sending the wounded first to a head/neck/spinal medical division near the front, then transferring them to a secondary station for eye care [94]. The measures succeeded. Early in the war, 69.7 percent of wounded eyes were treated by enucleation. By 1943, this figure was reduced to 37.7 percent [95]. Research continued at the Helmholtz Institute, mostly on trauma and wound healing. Other centers reported their studies of similar topics. Vladimir Filatov left Odessa in the occupied Ukraine in 1941, going first to Pjatigorsk, then to Tashkent. While his responsibilities were primarily clinical, even in Tashkent he maintained his research, resuming it in 1943 [96]. *Vestnik oftalmologii* carried studies on enucleation, splinters, foreign bodies, anesthesia, battlefield medicine, fractures, radiology, and infections. Other research was reported, but in considerably smaller volume on the subjects of color vision, optic physiology, lid cancer, tonometry, and vitamins. Trachoma doggedly persisted; reports of it appeared sporadically through the war years.

After the War, dedication to research and technology resumed, rising above its previous level. Filatov's Ukrainian Research Institute for Eye Diseases was rebuilt with sixteen laboratories (from eight), 300 beds (previously 200), and new outlying clinics in Stalino, Kherson, Pervomajsk, Vologda, and Sukhumi [97]. New machines and sciences allowed for new studies: electroretinography, used by A.I. Bogoslovskij and E.N. Semenovskaja; biochemistry, to study inner eye and anterior chamber acidity, the epithelium of the cornea, and polysaccharides by E. Zh. Tron, V.P. Roshchin, D.I. Berezinskoj, V.A. Vasiljev, and M.A. Rzajev; autoradiography, developed by D.S. Sivoshinskij and Ju. A. Belov; laser, studied by Chutko and Kerov in 1966; electron microscopy by L.F. Stebaev and R.S. Morozov; histochemistry by D.I. Antelov and P.S. Kapunovich; and many, many others [98]. The history of post-war Soviet ophthalmology is written more in terms of machines and methods than of men and women.

The official commitment to technology has been profound. Ophthalmologist-scientists such as M.M. Krasnov, who developed microsurgical techniques, have been honored with the Lenin Award [99]. Others have received the Stalin Award, the Order of Lenin, the Golden Star, or the Hero of Socialist Labor Award for scientific achievement. Interest in research has been intense in both medical and government circles. A report of the Academy of Medical Sciences of the USSR in 1983 noted: "The definition of a strategy of scientific medical research is the major task of the Academy as the cornerstone of medical science" [100]. Leonid Brezhnev, as president of the USSR, likewise noted in 1977, "In pondering the future, we ascribe great importance to science. It has to make an enormous contribution to the most important problems of building communism" [101]. He made his statement in conjunction with a report from the Central Committee of the Communist Party of the Soviet Union and the USSR Council of Ministers in 1978, "On Measures to Further Improve National Public Health," in which science was placed squarely at the base of solving the health problems of the nation.

Dedication to providing greater accessibility to service emerged in the post-war period. There were 63 departments of eye diseases in 1940; by 1967 there were 90. The number of eye specialists increased from 3212 to 13 146 in that time, and beds from 13015 to 35000 [102]. By 1962, trachoma dropped out as a significant cause of ocular morbidity in the Soviet Union. Recently, greater concern has been placed on myopia, estimated to afflict more than fifty million in the nation [103]. The Moscow Research Institute of Eye Microsurgery (the Helmholtz) has vigorously pursued treatment of this problem with the controversial operation, radial keratotomy.

In summary, ophthalmology in Russia developed from a Western, predominantly German, research-based tradition. It came to a nation with serious problems of eye disease. While providing medical service was a relatively low-status occupation in Russia, academia was not. Because of its scholarly roots, ophthalmology grew well in academia. As a specialty, it attracted people who aspired to accomplishment and action. As a science and a service, ophthalmology grew because of serious social need for adequate eye care, nurtured by its devoted cadre of well-placed, foreign-trained specialists. They met the need for eye care by staffing eye institutes, departments in universities, hospitals, and clinics, and by training community care eye doctors. While these ophthalmologists were not revolutionary in a political sense, they belonged to a tradition of social activism which was consistent with the policies of the new government in 1917. Moreover, they embraced something that was not only politically-safe, but politically-revered: research and technology. The advent of Soviet power was advantageous to ophthalmology in Russia because it gave the specialty more personnel and facilities to manage the formidable public health problems of trachoma, smallpox, glaucoma, and tuberculosis, and unconditional support for the development of research and technology. Given their specialty's heritage and endowment, ophthalmologists successfully traversed revolution, civil war, purges, world war, and technocracy.

Acknowledgements

This paper was prepared with the support of a grant from the National Endowment for the Humanities, tendered at the Kennedy Institute of Ethics, Georgetown University. The help of Daniel Fox, Edmund Pellegrino, Howard Carter, Mardi Patchell, Richard Caplan, Palmer Howard, Frederick Blodi, Steve Jones, and John Campano proved invaluable in its development.

Notes

1. B. Mironov, "Glasses for the Future," *Pravda*, 2/17/1983, p. 3.
2. George Gorin, *History of Ophthalmology*, Wilmington, Delaware: Publish or Perish, Inc., 1982. [English]
3. Anatoly Bezkorovainy, "Ophthalmologic Research in Pre-World I Russia," *Bulletin of the History of Medicine*, 1979, pp. 593–605. [English]
4. Hirschberg, *The History of Opthalmology*, Volume XII, translated by F.C. Blodi, J.P. Wayenborgh, Bonn (in press). [English]
5. Nancy Frieden, *Russian Physicians in an Era of Reform and Revolution, 1856–1905*, Princeton: Princeton University Press, 1981. [English]

6. Mark Field, *Soviet Socialized Medicine*, New York: The Free Press, 1967. [English]
7. Sergei Semjonovich Golovin, *On Blindness in Russia*, Odessa: Technique Press, 1910.
8. A. Ja. Saviotov, "Blindness in the USSR," *Vestnik oftalmologii*, 1932.
9. Vladimir Filatov, *My Path in Science*, Moscow: Foreign Language Publishers, 1957. [English translation]
10. Thomas Hall Shastid, *An Outline History of Ophthalmology*, Southridge, Massachusetts: American Optical Company, 1927. [English]
11. Frieden, p. 21.
12. Frieden, p. 22.
13. Frieden, p. 27.
14. Frieden, p. 30.
15. Frieden, pp. 67, 109.
16. Frieden, p. 83.
17. Hirschberg, p. 2.
18. V.A. Rukin, "Three Jubilee Dates in the History of Soviet Ophthalmology," *Oftalmologicheskij zhurnal*, v. 24, 1969, p. 627.
19. Hirschberg, p.109.
20. S.G. Magilnitskij, "First Experience with Russian Ophthalmologic Roentgenology in Eye Injuries," *Oftamologischeskij zhurnal*, v. 38, (2) 1983, p. 120.
21. Magilnitskij, "Roentgenology," p. 120.
22. Bezkorovainy, p. 599.
23. Bezkorovainy, p. 599.
24. S.G. Magilnitskij, "The First Antiglaucomatous Iridectomy in Russia," *Vestnik oftalmologii*, v. 80, (1) 1967, p. 85.
25. Bezkorovainy, p. 596.
26. Hirschberg, p. 68.
27. Hirschberg, p. 72.
28. P.G. Krasnikov, "An Outstanding Invention of a Russian Ophthalmologist," *Vestnik oftalmologii*, (6) 1984, p. 71.
29. Hirschberg, p. 75.
30. M.M. Krasnov, "Reminiscences of the Past: Adrian Aleksandrovich Kruikov, Editor of *Vestnik Oftalmologii* and Founder of the Moscow Ophthalmologic Society," *Vestnik oftalmologii*, (6) 1984), p. 5.
31. Gorin, P. 285.
32. Hirschberg, pp. 69–70.
33. V.D. Sutrin, "Herman Helmholtz and Ophthalmology," *Oftalmologicheskij zhurnal*, v. 30, (5) 1975, p. 391.
34. Hirschberg, p. 120.
35. Hirschberg, p. 119.
36. Hirschberg, p. 123.
37. Bezkorovainy, p. 604.
38. Hirschberg, p. 143.
39. Krasnikov, "Invention," p. 71.
40. Filatov, p. 1[illegible].
41. Rukin, p. 626.
42. Rukin, p. 626.
43. S.G. Magilnitskij, "The First Women Ophthalmologists in Southern Russia in the Nineteenth Century," *Oftalmologicheskij zhurnal*, v. 29, 1974, p. .74
44. Magilnitskij, "Women," p. 74.
45. N.I. Pirogov, *Sochinenija*, Kiev: Isdanie Pirogovskago T. V., 1910, p. 12.
46. Pirogov, *Sochinenija*, p. 3.
47. Frieden, p. 6.

48. cf. Pirogov, *Sochinenija*, eg p. 38, "Questions of Life."
49. P.G. Krasnikov, "S.S. Golovin," *Vestnik oftalmologii*, v. 79, 1966, p. 88.
50. Krasnikov, "Golovin," p. 89.
51. Krasnikov, "Golovin," p. 89.
52. Golovin, p. 1.
53. Golovin, p. 5.
54. Golovin, p. 17.
55. Golovin, pp. 17–18.
56. Golovin, pp. 24, 29.
57. Golovin, p. 45.
58. Golovin, p. 49.
59. Golovin, p. 77.
60. Golovin, p. 112.
61. P.G. Krasnikov, "L.G. Belliarminov – Outstanding Scientist, Public Figure, and Organizer of Ophthalmologic Care for the Population" *Vestnik oftalmologii*, (5) 1984, p. 69.
62. Krasnikov, "Belliarminov," p. 69.
63. Krasnikov, "Belliarminov," p. 69.
64. Krasnikov, "Belliarminov," p. 70.
65. Krasnikov, "Belliarminov," p. 70.
66. V.V. Volkov, "Military Ophthalmology in the Period of World War II," *Voenno-meditsinskij zhurnal*, (5) 1980, p. 50.
67. "A Distinguished Scientist and Ophthalmologist," *Oftalmologicheskij zhurnal*, v. 30, (1) 1979, p. 3.
68. Krasnikov, "Golovin," p. 89.
69. Filatov, in K.V. Trutneva, "Soviet Ophthalmology – Fifty Years," *Vestnik oftalmologii*, v. 80 (5) 1967, p. 7.
70. Vilatov, p. 141.
71. Bezkorovainy, p. 594.
72. Bezkorovainy, p. 594.
73. Frieden, p. 47.
74. S.G. Magilnitskij, "Ophthalmologists and Revolutionaries," *Vestnik oftalmologii*, (6) 1983, p. 73.
75. Magilnitskij, "Revolutionaries," p. 73.
76. Magilnitskij, "Revolutionaires," p. 73.
77. Magilnitskij, "Revolutionaries," p. 73.
78. Magilnitskij, "Revolutionaries," p. 73.
79. V.D. Timakov et al., "Medical Science," in I.P. Lidov (editor), *Sixty Years of Soviet Health*, Moscow: Medicine, 1977, p. 325.
80. Field, p. 175.
81. Trutneva, p. 7.
82. T.S. Kuznetsova et al., "Development of Medical Research Institutes," *Sovetskoe zdravokhranenie*, (12) 1982, p. 10.
83. Field, p. 177.
84. Kuznetsova, p. 10.
85. Trutneva, p. 8.
86. Trutneva, p. 8.
87. Saviotov, 1932.
88. Filatov, p. 17.
89. Filatov, p. 43.
90. Filatov, p. 43.
91. Trutneva, p. 8.
92. *Vestnik oftalmologii* of these years.

93. E.F. Levkoeva et al., "The History of the Department of Pathologic Anatomy and History of the Moscow Research Institute of Eye Disease in Memory of Helmholtz," *Arkhiv patologii*, v. 39, 1977, p. 86.
94. Volkov, p. 50.
95. Volkiov, p. 53.
96. Filatov, p. 11.
97. Filatov, p. 12.
98. E.I. Kovalevskij, "Soviet Ophthalmology (on the 50th Anniversary of the USSR)," *Vestnik oftalmologii*, (6) 1972, p. 5.
99. "Lenin's Principles in the Practice of Ophthalmologists," *Vestnik oftalmologii*, (3) 1980, p. 5.
100. N.I. Bochkov, "The 47th Session of the General Meeting of the Academy of Medical Sciences of the USSR," *Vestnik Akademii meditsinskikh Nauk CCCP*, (19) 1983, p. 5.
101. Leonid Brezhnev, in *Pravda*, 11/2/77, p. 2, from G.I. Siderenko, "On the Work of the Presidium of the Academy of Medical Sciences of the USSR," *Vestnik Akademii meditsinskikh Nauk CCCP*, (1) 1979, p. 4.
102. Trutneva, p. 8.
103. Mironov, p. 3.

Source of Figs. 1–4: Hirschberg, J., "Geschichte der Augenheilkunde: Die Augenärzte Rußlands, 1800–1875". In: Graefe-Saemisch, *Handbuch der Gesamten Augenheilkunde*, Drittes Buch, Siebzehnter Abschnitt, Kapitel 23. Berlin, Julius Springer, 1915–1918.

References

[All sources are IN RUSSIAN except as noted.]

Bezkorovainy A. Ophthalmologic research in Pre-World I Russia. Bulletin of the History of Medicine 1979; 593–605 [English].

Bochkov NI. The 47th session of the general meeting of the Academy of Medical Sciences of the USSR. Vestnik Akademii meditsinskikh Nauk CCCP 1983; 19: 4–11.

Brzheskij VChi. Ophthalmologists in the peoples memory. Vestnik oftalmologii 1979; 6: 61–2.

Chernukh AM et al. Raising the effectiveness of priority research in scientific institutions of the Academy of Medical Sciences of the USSR. Vestnik Akademii meditsinskikh Nauk SSSR 1980; 4: 22–28.

On the distant development of fundamental research for medicine. Vestnik Akademii meditsinskikh Nauk SSSR. 1981; 4: 100–106.

A distinguished scientist and ophthalmologist. Oftalmolgicheskij zhurnal, v. 30 1979; 1: 306.

Field M. Soviet socialized medicine. New York: The Free Press, 1967 [English].

Filatov VP. My path in science. Moscow: Foreign Language Publishers, 1957 [English translation].

Frieden N. Russian Physicians in an era of reform and revolution, 1856–1905. Princeton: Princeton University Press, 1981 [English].

Glovin SS. On blindness in Russia. Odessa: Technique Press, 1910.

Gorin G. History of ophthalmology. Wilmington, Delaware: Publish or Perish Inc, 1982 [English].

Hirschberg J. The history of ophthalmology, Volume XII, translated by Blodi FC, JP Wayenborgh. Bonn (in press) [English].

Kovalevskij EI. Soviet ophthalmology (on the 50th anniversary of the USSR). Vestnik oftalmologii 1972; 6: 3–9.

Krasnikov PG. L.G. Belliarminov – Outstanding scientist, public figure, and organizer of ophthalmologic care for the population. Vestnik oftalmologii 1984; 5: 69–70.

Krasnikov PG. S.S. Golovin. Vestnik oftalmologii, v. 79. 1966; 11–12.

Krasnikov PG. An outstanding invention of a Russian ophthalmologist. Vestnik oftalmologii 1984; 6: 70–72.

Krasnov MM. Reminiscences of the past: Adrian Aleksandrovich Kruikov, Editor of Vestnik oftalmologii and Founder of the Moscow Ophthalmologic Society. Vestnik oftalmologii. 1984; 6: 4–6.

Kuznetsova TS et al. Development of medical research institutes. Sovetskoe zdravokhranenie. 1982; 12: 10.

Lebekhov PI. The 100th anniversary of postgraduate training of eye doctors. Vestnik oftalmologii v. 101, 1985; 5: 71–72.

Levkoeva EF et al. The history of the Department of Pathologic Anatomy and history of the Moscow Research Institute of Eye Disease in memory of Helmholtz. Arkhiv patologii, v. 39, 1977; 84–88.

Lenin's principles in the practice of ophthalmologists. Vestnik oftalmologii. 1980; 3: 3–5.

Ljubchenko IA. 150th anniversary of the Moscow City Eye Clinic. Vestnik oftalmologii 1977; 1: 85–86..

Magilnitskij SG. The first antiglaucomatous iridectomy in Russia. Vestnik oftalmologii, v. 80, 1967; 1: 85–86.

Magilnitskij SG. First experience with Russian ophthalmologic roentgenology in eye injuries. Oftalmologischeskij zhurnal, v. 38, 1983; 2: 119–120.

Magilnitskij SG. The first women ophthalmologists in Southern Russia in the nineteenth century. Oftalmologicheskij zhurnal, v. 29, 1974; 73–76.

Magilnitskij SG. Ophthalmologists and revolutionaries. Vestnik oftalmologii. 1983; 6: 72–75.

Mironov V. Glasses for the future. Pravda 2/17/1983; 3.

Pastore N. Selective history of theories of visual perception: 1650–1950. New York: Oxford University Press, 1971.

Pirogov NI. Sevastopol Letters. St. Petersburg: M. Merkushev, 1907.

Pirogov NI. Sochinenija. Kiev: Izdanie Pirogovskago T. Va., 1910.

Rukin VA. Three jubilee dates in the history of Soviet ophthalmology. Oftalmolgischeskij zhurnal, v. 24, 1969; 625–627.

Saviotov AJa. Blindness in the USSR. Vestnik oftalmologii, 1932.

Shastid TH. An outline history of ophthalmology. Southridge, Massachusetts: American Optical Company, 1927 [English].

Siderenko GI. On the work of the presidium of the Academy of Medical Sciences of the USSR. Vestnik Akademii meditsinskikh Nauk CCCP 1979; 1: 3–14.

Sutrin VD. Herman Helmholtz and ophthalmology. Oftamologicheskij zhurnal, v. 30, 1975; 5: 390–391.

Timakov VD et al. Medical science. In: IP Lidov, ed. Sixty years of Soviet health. Moscow: Medicine, 1977.

Trutneva KV. Soviet ophthalmology – fifty years. Vestnik oftalmologii, v. 80 1967; 5: 7–12.

Volkov VV et al. Military ophthalmology in the period of World War II. Voenno-meditsinskij zhurnal 1980; 5: 50–53.

Address for offprints: Henry J. Carson, M.D., 3161 North Cambridge Street, Chicago, IL 60657, USA.

Documenta Ophthalmologica 71: 195–201, 1989.

The founding of the First University Eye Clinic in Vienna

HELMUT FANTA
Vienna, Austria

The First University Eye Clinic in Vienna, the first of its kind in the world, is closely connected with the name Georg Joseph Beer (1763–1821).

In the 18th century eye doctors in Europe were either general practitioners or surgeons. In Vienna they were mostly anatomists. At the same time, in many European countries, lectures in ophthalmology were prepared but seldom held, mostly because of lack of interest. Rivals from other branches of medicine also obstructed these lectures.

In contrast to other branches of medicine, ophthalmology achieved its autonomy relatively early in Vienna.

The Empress Maria Theresia (who reigned from 1740 to 1780) was interested in creating a modern faculty of medicine. For this reason she asked her personal physician, Van Swieten, who had studied under Boerhaave, to reorganize the hospitals and the medical faculty. At that time the University of Vienna had no eye clinic. There were only some small private eye hospitals. Such small eye hospitals could be found all over Europe during the second half of the 18th century.

Van Swieten was aware of the advantages of a cataract extraction and studied the operation with Daviel in Paris as early as 1751. Palluci, an Italian eye doctor, was called to Vienna and he attempted to settle in Vienna, but without success.

In the 18th century there were many itinerant eye doctors who operated, mostly cataracts, as they travelled from city to city. Dr. de Wenzel of Paris, the best cataract surgeon in Europe after Daviel's death, was invited to Vienna to operate on one of the Empress' ladies-in-waiting. He received 10 000 florins as a fee (about $100 000 U.S. dollars). De Wenzel was asked to train other surgeons and for this he received a salary. His students were not taught the details of the cataract operation and for this reason de Wenzel had to be called back.

Later Joseph Barth (1745–1818)(Fig. 1), an anatomist, finally learned the operative technique so well that he earned a reputation as an excellent eye surgeon. A decree on October 23, 1773 made Barth lecturer in ophthalmology besides his main obligations as an anatomist, but he had neither a clinic

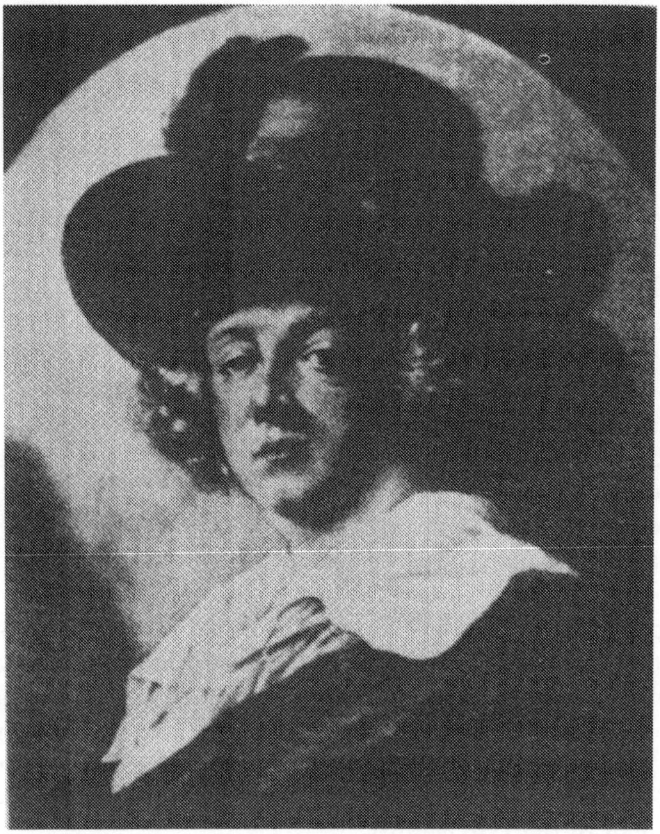

Fig. 1. Joseph Barth.

nor a hospital. In 1791 he resigned from his teaching post at the Vienna university.

His successor was the physiologist Georg Prohaska (1749–1820), who gave lectures in ophthalmology combined with advanced anatomy. It was especially Prohaska who attempted to prevent the foundation of an eye clinic.

The first great teacher of international renown was Georg Joseph Beer (1763–1821)(Fig. 2).

Beer was born in 1763 and was meant to become a priest. He first attended the Vienna Academy of Arts, which turned out to be an asset for his teaching activities. He painted beautiful and accurate pictures of eye diseases which he used for student instructions.

He first learned some ophthalmology when studying anatomy. He graduated as a medical doctor in 1786. After his graduation he remained in

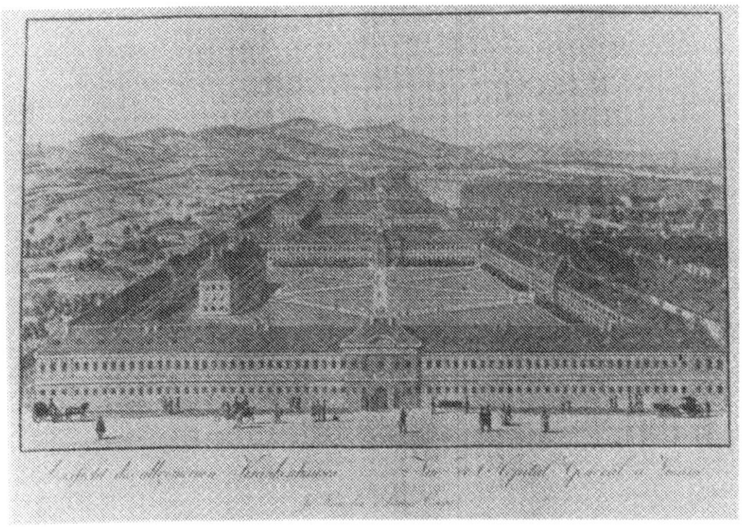

Fig. 2. Georg Joseph Beer.

the anatomical institute. The head of this institute was Barth, who was also an ophthalmologist. Beer was an able assistant of Barth at all operations, however, he was hindered by Barth in all his ophthalmological activities. Beer left Barth and became a general practitioner. At this time he was already interested in ophthalmology and established an eye practice where he treated poor people free of charge.

Later he founded a private clinic for rich and poor alike, but wealthy patients were till the end of the 19th century operated on at home. Beer's private clinic was transformed into a public hospital in 1806. Beer's untiring diligence, his initiative and action, his systematic teaching and his skill as a surgeon and teacher were the foundation stones of the Viennese school of ophthalmology.

It was due to Beer that the intracapsular cataract extraction became later the method of choice. Before that this method had been known, but not practiced, as it demanded a special technique. Significantly better results, however, were obtained by this method. In his book about this technique one can read that the recovery is faster, the visual acuity is better and there is no secondary cataract (1799). He also described an operation to form a new pupil in the case that the pupil is pulled up after a cataract operation or after injuries.

His experience was collected in several books. In addition to a textbook for ophthalmology, he wrote many monographs on operative techniques and the treatment of various eye diseases. He also wrote a book for the general public on eye care. The title: *The Eye – or the Attempt to Protect the Most Noble Gift of Creation from the Extremely Ruinous Influence of Our Age.*

This book appeared in 1800 and 1813 in Vienna and 1807 in French and also in Polish. This was a humorous and skillful presentation of his oculistic health rules for lay readers.

In his textbook one can find excellent pictures of pathologic changes of the eye, which were drawn by himself.

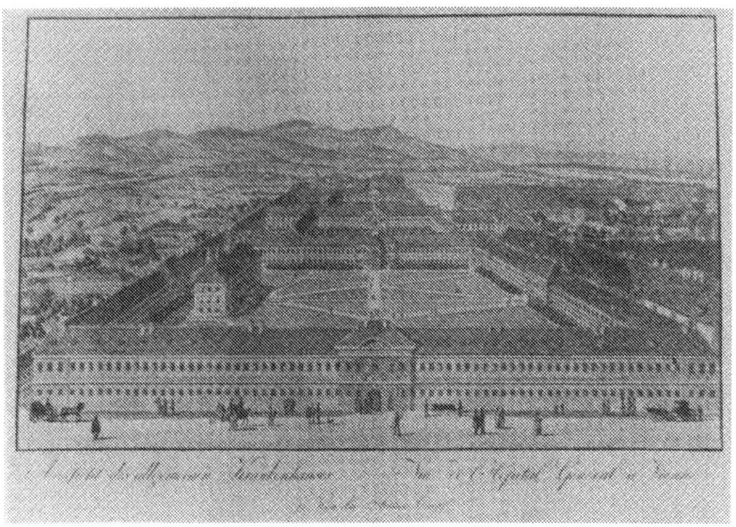

Fig. 3. The general hospital in Vienna.

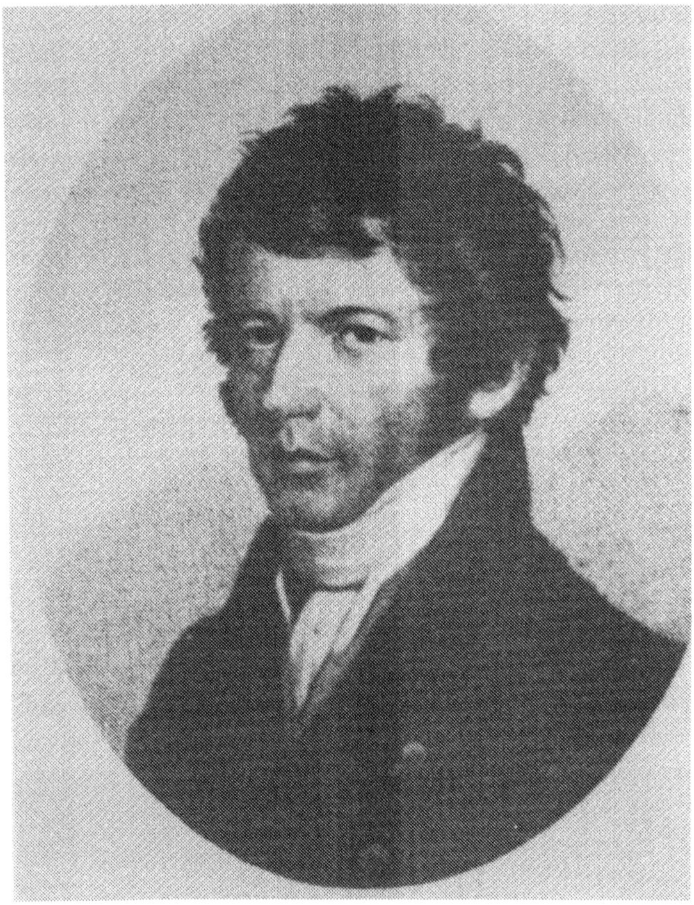

Fig. 4. Friedrich Jäger.

In 1805 and 1807 he suggested that the government build a university eye clinic, but his rivals from other hospitals in the city prevented it. After a long struggle against his contemporary university colleagues, Beer at last achieved the establishment of a university eye clinic and on 28th April 1812 he began his lectures "*Practical and Theoretical Ophthalmology*"; this is the date of the foundation of the first university eye clinic in the world. In the big central hospital called "*Allgemeines Krankenhaus*" he was given beds and an operating theater. Even today one of the Viennese eye clinics, The First University Eye Clinic, is still in the same place, but much bigger (Fig. 3).

Unfortunately, Beer could enjoy this achievement only for a few years because he had an apoplectic attack in 1819 and died in 1821.

Beer achieved everything he had striven for in his life. For the Viennese medical faculty it was a great loss that he died so soon after his appointment. He wanted his student and son-in-law, Friedrich Jaeger, to become his successor, but Anton Rosas was selected instead. Rosas was the head of the University Eye Clinic in Vienna from 1821 until 1855 when he was followed by Arlt.

Friedrich Jaeger (Fig. 4) and his son, Eduard Jaeger, established the tradition of the Viennese school in eye surgery. Friedrich Jaeger was the head of the eye department of the military academy "*Josephinum*" until 1848 and died in 1872.

Friedrich Jaeger operated with skill and accuracy for many years. He modified the cataract incision (Fig. 5). It was a new method which decreased the loss of eyes from 10% to 4.5%. Many young eye doctors from all over the world came to Vienna to learn Jaeger's method. He did not publish all his techniques, though his students asked him to do so. On the urgent request of von Graefe he made drawings of his observations which he later published.

In 1825 he was sent to Klagenfurt, in the southern Austrian province of Carinthia, to treat the Egyptian eye disease which had broken out in the army. He recognized it as a contagious disease and isolated the afflicted

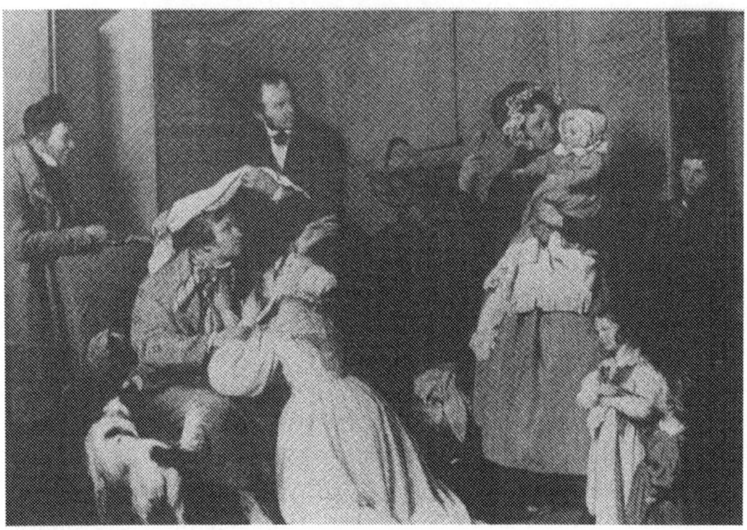

Fig. 5. Friedrich Jäger is depicted in this painting by Josef Danhauser called "*Der Augenarzt*" 1837 (Histor. Museum der Stadt Wien).

soldiers. He introduced copper sulfate treatment with great success. When I was a young doctor we still used the copper stick in the clinic before the introduction of sulfonamides. An exact description of trachoma was his only literary output.

Sultan Mohammed II from Turkey asked Jaeger to set up a medical school in Galata Serail. Galata Serail is now the central part of Istanbul. For many years members of the military academy "*Josephinum*" worked in the Turkish medical school to train students in ophthalmology. After 1848 he was active only in his private practice and his private hospital. He was knighted with the Order of the Iron Crown and received the title "*Von Jaxthal.*"

His son, Eduard von Jaeger, continued his work in Vienna. Jaeger's student, Piringer, worked for a long time in Graz.

The tradition of the Vienna Ophthalmological School can be followed during the next decades. It was always characterized by the high standard of diagnosis and surgical treatment. The University Eye Clinic was soon too small for the Viennese population so in the immediate vicinity hospitals with eye departments were founded which were directed by excellent heads.

Nevertheless, it was necessary to set up a *Second University Eye Clinic* which was done in 1883 and Eduard von Jaeger (1818–1884) was its first head, but only for one year.

Ferdinand Arlt (1812–1887) and Ernst Fuchs (1851–1930) were teachers who held up the international reputation of the Vienna Ophthalmological School before the First World War.

Address for offprints: Prof. Dr. Helmut Fanta, Ferstelgasse 4, A-1090 Vienna, Austria.

Documenta Ophthalmologica 71: 203–204, 1989.

Short communication

The Lisbon Institute of Ophthalmology – Instituto de Oftalmologia Dr. Gama Pinto – its founding and history

J. RIBEIRO DA SILVA
Instituto de Oftalmologia Dr. Gama Pinto, Travessa Larga 2, 1100 Lisbon, Portugal

The Lisbon Institute of Ophthalmology, belonging to the Lisbon University, was organized in 1885 by Prof. Gama Pinto, the first chairman of ophthalmology of the Portuguese Universities (Fig. 1).

Gama Pinto, studied Medicine in Lisbon and Ophthalmology in Heidelberg with Otto Becker. In the Heidelberg University he became Privat Docent, at the time of Otto Becker.

In 1885, Gama Pinto returned to Portugal with the intention to organize and to create in Lisbon an Institute of Ophthalmology, which he did with the help and understanding of King Louis I.

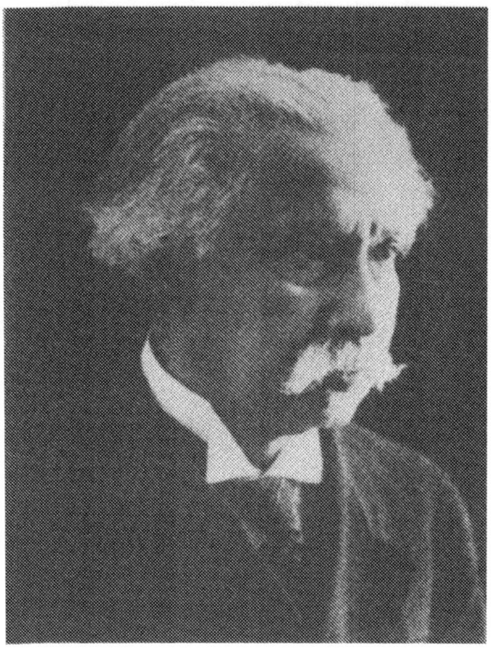

Fig. 1. Portrait of Dr. Gama Pinto. Private collection. Lisbon Institute of Ophthalmology.

The Institute appeared in Lisbon in 1888, exactly one hundred years ago.

At the beginning, the Institute was localized in a Palace from the 17th century, Palácio Penamacor, where part of the Institute still remains.

In the beginning of the 20th Century another building appeared connected with the old Palace and in this building a modern Hospital and an Institute, since then developed.

After Gama Pinto there were four Directors of the Lisbon Institute, Prof. Borges de Sousa, one of Gama Pinto's pupils, the ophthalmologist who brought to Portugal the surgery of retinal detachment, Prof. Lopes de Andrade who did very important scientific work on the trachoma in Portugal. Prof. Almeida Lima pupil of the Portuguese Nobel Prize, Prof. Egas Moniz who developed in Portugal neuro-ophthalmology and Prof. Ribeiro da Silva, the present Director.

The Lisbon Institute of Ophthalmology has a very interesting technological and historical Museum of Portuguese Ophthalmology.

The Lisbon Institute of Ophthalmology has a journal, the Portuguese Archives of Ophthalmology.

The most important scientific works since Gama Pinto are connected with ocular pathology, viral infections, electrophysiology of the visual system, particularly the studies of the V.E.P. and microsurgery of the eye. It is interesting to remember that in 1900 Gama Pinto wrote a very important book on glaucoma, translated at that time into French and published also in the French Encyclopedia of Ophthalmology.

It is also very interesting to remember that the Institute is pioneer in the electrophsyiological studies of the visual system; particularly the research on the VEP, research that started in Lisbon in 1954.

Address for offprints: Prof. Dr. Ribeiro da Silva, Instituto de Oftalmologia Dr. Gama Pinto, Travessa Larga 2, 1100 Lisbon, Portugal.

Documenta Ophthalmologica 71: 205–219, 1989.

Field Marshall Radetzky's orbital abscess

FREDERICK C. BLODI
Department of Ophthalmology, University of Iowa, Iowa City, IA 52242, USA

Past history

On October 9, 1840, Field Marshal Radetzky (Fig. 1) supervised the annual fall maneuvers of the Austrian Army in northern Italy (Fig. 2). The maneuvers that year were held in Castiglione delle Stiviere in Lombardy, a small town close to Brescia and the Lago di Garda, only 25 miles northwest of the famous fortress of Mantova. The Field Marshall was at that time 75 years old, but in excellent health. As a lifelong soldier, he was a vigorous man who was in complete control of the situation. He was the commanding general of the relatively recently established Lombardo-Venetian Kingdom, a crownland of Austria governed by Viceroy Archduke Rainer.

Radetzky enjoyed the annual maneuvers. After all, he had introduced the modern concept of these exercises, had delineated their objectives and described their logistics. He had published a number of papers and a whole monograph on this topic. He was the world expert in this field. A number of spectators and observers were present, among them Alexander II, Czar of Russia, representatives of the neighboring and allied duchies of Tuscany, Parma and Modena, as well as officers representing Bavaria, England, France, Holland, Spain, Sweden and Switzerland. The Field Marshall, the "military schoolmaster of Europe," obviously put on a good show.

But it had been a hard day. It was unusually hot for this time of the year and Radetzky had been on his horse for more than five hours. The sun beat down on him and his face became red, he experienced a severe right frontal headache, his temperature rose and the right eye started to protrude.

The Field Marshall had in the past had only minor health problems, but he had experienced a similar attack two years earlier in 1839 while reviewing a gathering of the troops near Pordenone, about 50 miles north of Venice.

He had for years been under the treatment of his good friend, Dr. Christoph Hartung, Imperial Royal Counselor and Directing Staff Physi-

This paper is dedicated to the memory of my teacher and friend, Prof. Dr. J. Böck, erstwhile head of the II. University Eye Clinic in Vienna, who supported my interest in this topic and obtained valuable source material for me.

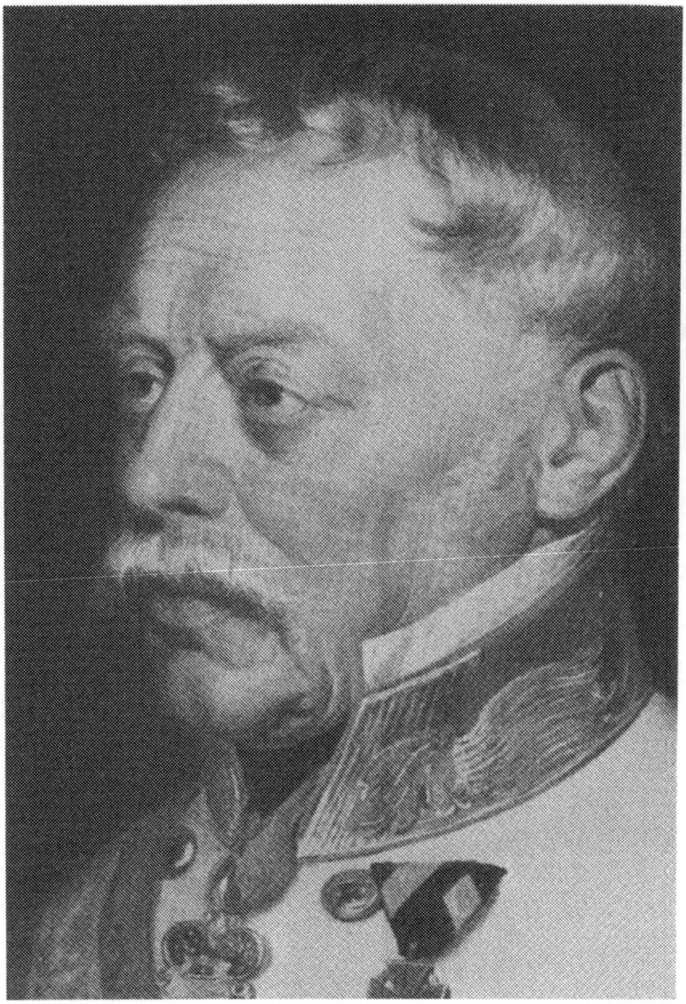

Fig. 1. Radetzky as commander-in-chief of the army in the Lombardo-Venetian Kingdom.

cian of the Army in the Kingdom. The Field Marshall did not mind that Dr. Hartung was a homeopathic physician, a disciple of Samuel Christoph Hahnemann (1755–1843), who claimed that "similia similibus curentur." This notion that a drug which at toxic levels produced a certain effect, seizures, for example, could be used in very small doses to defend the body against the same effect ("the law of similars") was very popular at that time. It was claimed that solutions of less than one in a million were still therapeutically effective.

During the first half of the 19th century, allopaths and homeopaths went

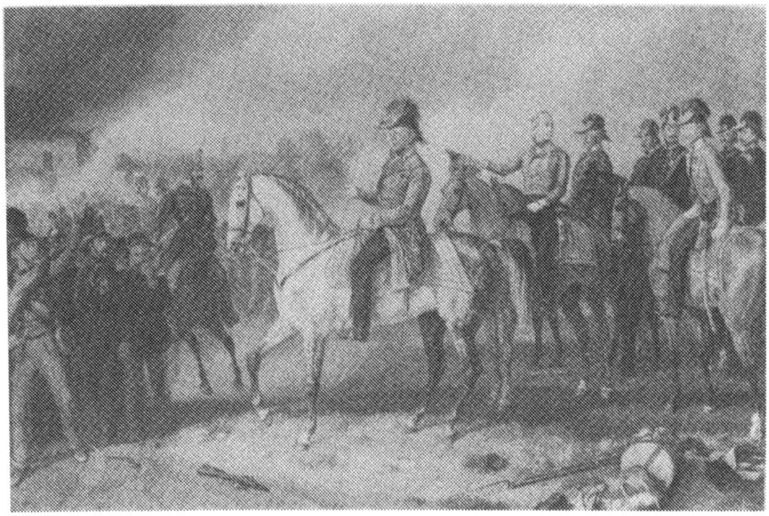

Fig. 2. Radetzky entering Milan (painting by Albrecht Adam).

to the same schools, had the same graduate training and acquired the same academic degrees. During postgraduate training, they split into two camps, but still belonged to the same medical societies and academies. However, there was no love lost between the two groups and they fought continuously.

Present illness

The next day the eye condition improved. Radetzky spent again six hours on his horse reviewing a church parade of the army.

During the following weeks his eye seemed to wax and wane, but the right eye remained constantly injected; a tumefaction developed at the nasal canthus, the lower lid remained swollen and the patient complained about tearing. The Field Marshall spent a few weeks in Verona, visited Modena and returned in December to his headquarters in Milan. The condition had taken a definite turn for the worse. Dr. Hartung became concerned. He diagnosed a fungus of the right orbit and put the patient on systemic medications to confine the fungus and to improve the patient's resistance. He prescribed ten different compounds, all in the most minute concentrations.

Dr. Hartung kept detailed notes on the course of the disease. Each week he sent a report to Vienna to Count Ignaz Hardegg-Glatz und im Marchfeld, Court War Counselor (Minister of War). These notes were later published [1].

Consultations

In January Professor Flarer of Pavia was called in consultation. Francisco Flarer (1791–1859) was born in Meran in southern Tyrol, studied in Innsbruck and Landshut, graduating in Pavia in 1815. He worked with Beer in Vienna and became a good friend of F. Jaeger. In 1819 he was appointed professor at the University of Pavia, succeeding Antonio Scarpa and Tommaso Volpi.

Flarer arrived in Milan on January 7, 1841 and saw the patient immediately. According to Hartung, Flarer thought that nothing could be done and prescribed corrosive mercury sublimate, one drop every morning. Flarer saw the patient once more on the following morning and again maintained that no cure was possible, only a palliative treatment could be given and no suitable medication was available.

The fungus kept on growing; the tumour was eight lines (about 16 mm) wide; ocular motility was reduced, but vision was good. There developed a spongy, pale red, nontender, granulated, elastic tumefaction between the inner canthus and the globe.

The news reached Vienna and the court became concerned. The emperor wrote on January 18, 1841 to Count Hardegg: "... I desire to give a proof to the field Marshall and to my army how much I am concerned about the health of the Marshall that I have sent without delay the professor of ophthalmology at the Joseph-Academy, staff physician Friedrich Jaeger to Milan for consultation" [2].

Jaeger arrived in Milan on January 25 and saw the patient the following day. Flarer and Hartung were also present. Jaeger thought there was no cure and an operation would not help. Jaeger called it a dyscrasia. Flarer mentioned a scirrhus, turning into cancer.

Jaeger stayed for four days, informed the viceroy and allegedly told Radetzky to "trust Hartung."

Course of the disease

During the following months the condition improved gradually on homeopathic treatment. There was copious secretion, but the swelling decreased. On April 19, the birthday of the emperor, the Field Marshall had a strenuous day with a long church service, military parade and reception, but he felt fine, wore no patch and considered himself cured.

Hartung now evaluated the various medications he had used. Arsenic and psorin made the condition worse; there was some improvement on herpetin and considerable success with carbo animalis. The best results were obtained with Thuja occidentalis. This tree extract was diluted (one drop in 3 ounces of water) and given orally 1 tablespoon 3 times a day for 3 days, then 6 drops in 4 ounces of water for 5 days; it was also used externally. Hartung then added carbo animalis and gave the two medications alternatingly or together.

The patient felt restored, worked and travelled a great deal. The right eye still teared easily.

Hartung ended his notes on June 12, 1849 with the triumphant statement that homeopathy had healed an incurable disease.

The news travels

The news of this miraculous cure of a severe eye condition affecting the most famous soldier of his time travelled fast and kept all of Europe humming. Many homeopaths claimed now that Thuja could cure cancer. Griesselich, a German homeopathic physician, first expressed some words of doubt. He brought up the question of dosage and type of medication. Arsenic, which Hartung had tried first, aggravated the exophthalmus; psorine was then used, but it enlarged the fungus; carbo animalis had little effect. As none of these was useful, Hartung tried Thuja (which he had also successfully used for tonsilitis, exanthema and scirrhus of the nipples and Hahnemann had recommended it against the stye). This seemed successful; but why was then after eight days carbo animalis added? Why was this necessary if Thuja was curative?

Griesselich asked the question whether a dilution down to 1:10 million really is more than water [3]. Has the dosage not been diluted down to nothing, he asks. We only lose time with such infinitesimal dilutions. Local applications should be preferred, as they avoid the detour through the stomach.

Ludwig Griesselich was born 1804 in Baden and died 1848 in Prussia. He was an excellent botanist, became a military physician and a homeopath. He tried hard to elevate the standards of homeopathy fighting exaggerations and disclaiming miraculous cures. Such homeopaths, he said, are not our colleagues. They resemble God, making something out of nothing. Though he had worked with Hahnemann in Köthen, he later attacked the latter's famous book "Chronische Krankheiten." Griesselich was for many years the editor of the homeopathic journal "Hygea."

In two anonymous articles [4, 5] more questions were raised and the affair was covered with ridicule. The author (Griesselich?) said that Radetzky for three years had been unsuccessfully treated by the homeopath Hartung and that he had swallowed more homeopathic pills than he fired bullets. He went on to say that during the consultation Flarer was ordered *not* to remove the dressing, except when Hartung was present, but Hartung could not be found; Flarer had to return frustrated to Pavia.

In the second article [5] the author (Griesselich?) again discussed the question: "If the homeopathic medication was so wonderful and curative, why did it not work during the preceding three years while the Field Marshall was being treated by Dr. Hartung? Why was the treatment only effective after consultation with Professor Flarer?" Flarer had prescribed $\frac{1}{4}$ grain of mercury chloride daily. The patient took it for 12 days until Jaeger arrived who agreed with the treatment and added sublimate. Shortly thereafter the eye improved miraculously.

All these attacks were answered in a monograph which appeared anonymously 1843 in Munich [6]. Part I contains the whole history of the disease as recorded by Hartung and is not essentially different from the description given in reference 1, but occasionally amplified and full of self-aggrandizement and justifications.

Part II is a letter allegedly written by Radetzky to a Viennese newspaper, the "Wiener Zeitung," dated May 12, 1841. In it the writer thanks the homeopathic physician Dr. Hartung for curing his eye disease, which others had thought to be lethal. This letter never appeared in the paper. Its authenticity is dubious.

Part III reprints reference 4 and declares it full of defamation and lies, as it is void of proofs and scientific arguments. The author wonders how such a vulgar article could have been printed in a scientific journal.

Part IV brings Dr. Hartung's answers to the publication quoted in part III. It brings a testimonial written by Radetzky on April 4, 1842 in Milan verifying the fact that Hartung had saved his life. It also contains a thank-you note to Hartung from Countess v. Werkheim, the Field Marshall's daughter (Milan, May 17, 1841).

Part V is a postscript by Hartung and contains mainly rebuttals to various comments and footnotes which appeared in the Allgemeine Zeitung f. Chirurgie.

The debate

The news of Radetzky's miraculous cure was discussed and argued in many professional societies and learned academies. Nowhere was the discussion more vehement and vitriolic than in the Belgian Royal Academy of Medicine – at least no other debate was so thoroughly reported and published [7].

The violent discussion started innocently enough with a presentation by Cartier [8] on the cholera epidemic. Varlez, a homeopathic physician in the audience, interrupted the speaker. He wanted to emphasize the value of highly diluted medications and drew attention to Hartung's success in treating a fungus-like eye tumor of Field Marshall Radetzky with homeopathic medications.

Fallot [9] answered Varlez by quoting Griesselich [3] who maintained that only the topical applications of a drug to the affected organ were useful. The internal administration of medications in minimal concentrations was superfluous. Infinitesimal doses, he said, only led to loss of time.

Varlez [10] returned to his accusations and bet 20 000 francs for the benefit of the poor of Brussels if anybody could find in that issue of the Annales d'oculistique [3] what Fallot had claimed and maintained. He quoted Hartung who said that the disease thought to be incurable had been healed by homeopathic treatment.

Varlez had written to Petroz (who had translated Hartung's report [1]), who answered him on October 1, 1849 asserting that homeopathy had cured the Marshall. Griesselich – who was now dead – had argued only against the dose used, not against the principle of the homeopathic treatment. Varlez also contacted Roth (the second translator of Hartung's report [1]) who assured him also that homeopathy had cured the Marshall.

Varlez now presented the history and findings claiming that Hartung of Milan cured the patient with homeopathic doses of carbo animalis and Thuja. Radetzky had confirmed this in a letter to Varlez of December 13, 1849.

Fallot [11] answered accusing Varlez of defamation; he reported that the second anonymous report [5] was actually written by Dr. Gaal. There were interruptions and catcalls. It was claimed that Griesselich did *not* find the homeopathic treatment successful. Varlez finally lost his bet. Radetzky's statement was nothing more than a solicited testimonial – the kind that charlatans are particularly fond of.

Dramatis personae

It is interesting to examine what influence this episode had on the lives of the main participants of our dissertation.

The *patient* himself seems to have remained calm and collect. There is no evidence that he took a prolonged sick leave. Once his eye had improved, he spent a few weeks in Verona, but even there he kept on working and soon returned to his headquarters in Milan. For him this was a minor affair.

The definitive biography of Radetzky [12] is an encyclopedic tome with 555 pages, 440 footnotes and references, 10 pages of pertinent bibliography and a list of all of Radetzky's publications, yet it gives only one paragraph (on page 217) to this eye disease. More recent biographies do not mention the episode at all [13].

Radetzky (1766–1858) came from a family of Austrian military men. He was born near Prague and served under five emperors. He participated in the war against the Turks, against France and especially in the campaigns against Napoleon. He was chief of the general staff under Prince Schwarzenberg at the Battle of the Nations near Leipzig (1813) when Napoleon's power was finally broken. He rose rapidly in rank and in 1836 became field marshall, the highest ranking officer in the Austrian army.

He wrote numerous articles, manuals and books on strategy, weaponry and logistics. His bravery earned him the highest orders.

But his greatest triumphs were yet to come. The revolution of 1848 involved not only Paris and Vienna, Berlin and Dresden, but also northern Italy, especially Milan and Venice. Here the fight for freedom and democracy was combined with a desire of the Italian people for independence and unity. In that respect the Kingdom of Piedmont was their hope. Radetzky (Fig. 3) crushed them completely thereby saving the Austrian empire and the House of Hapsburg. After the Battle of Novara (1949) Carlo Alberto Savoy-Carignan, King of Sardinia, had to abdicate in favor of his son, Vittorio Emanuele II.

With Prince Eugene of Savoy and Archduke Karl, Radetzky became the most famous hero of Austria. He has been honored in many poems, novels and plays. Most famous is Grillparzer's [14] line: "In your camp is Austria." Best known all over the world is a piece of music, the Radetzky March by Johann Strauss, Sr. (1849).

In 1849, at the age of 83 (Fig. 4), Radetzky became Governor General of the Kingdom of Lombardy-Venetia. He resigned 1857 (Fig. 5).

He is buried at the unusual open-air pantheon on the Danube (Fig. 6). Among the many monuments dedicated to him, the one in Vienna is the grandest. It is by Kaspar von Zambusch (1892) and stands on the Ring in front of the old War Ministry (Fig. 7).

He has become a folk hero, referred to as "Papa Radetzky" and is better known than the five emperors whom he served.

Hartung graduated from the University of Vienna in 1812 and soon became an enthusiastic homeopath. In 1833 he was appointed Chief Medical Officer of the Austrian Army in northern Italy. After curing the Field Marshall, Hartung became famous and many patients sought his advice. He died in Baden near Vienna [15].

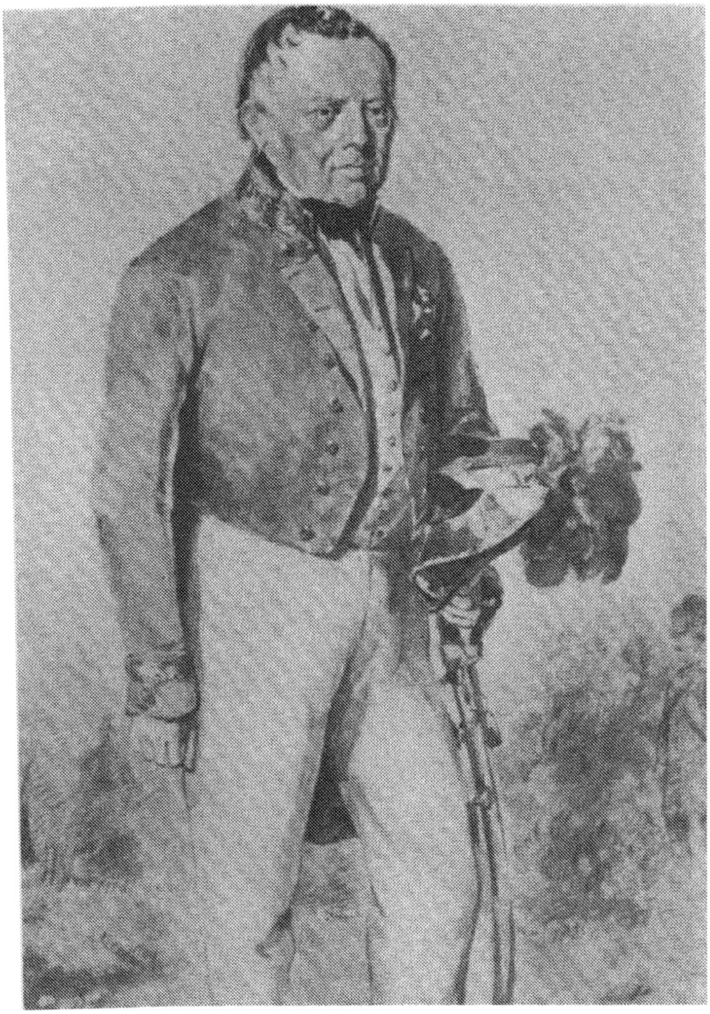

Fig. 3. Radetzky in Milan in 1848 (watercolor by Skallitzky).

Of course, all homeopaths were most thankful to Hartung. He had made them respectable and all over Europe they became more aggressive and confident.

Samuel Hahnemann, the German physician and founder of homeopathy, who lived his last years in Paris sent Hartung a portrait engraved into carnelian quartz which was later set in a ring and has been passed on from one generation of homeopaths to the next.

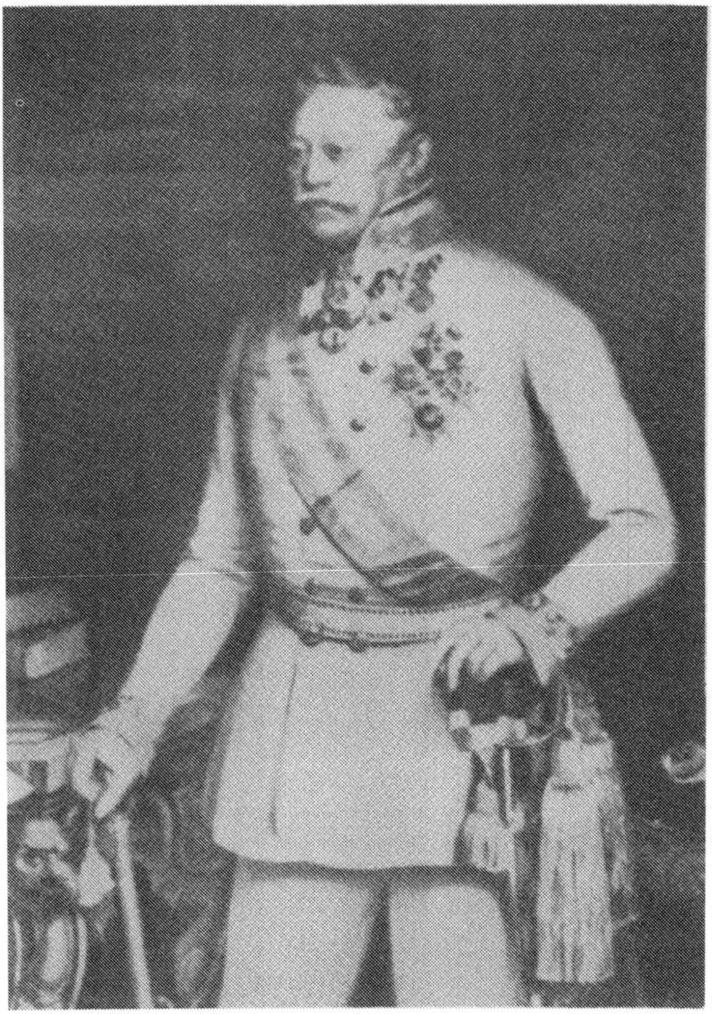

Fig. 4. Radetzky as Governor General in 1850 (oil painting by Eduard Klieber).

Francisco *Flarer* was for forty years chairman of the Department of Ophthalmology in Pavia. He was a representative of the old school, preferred couching cataracts to extracting them and recommended a hair rope (seton) inserted into the anterior chamber as a treatment of corneal staphyloma [16]. On the other hand, he was one of the first to give an excellent description of iritis.

Flarer was obviously embarrassed about the notoriety of Radetzky's homeopathic cure. In order to set the record straight he wrote on April 28,

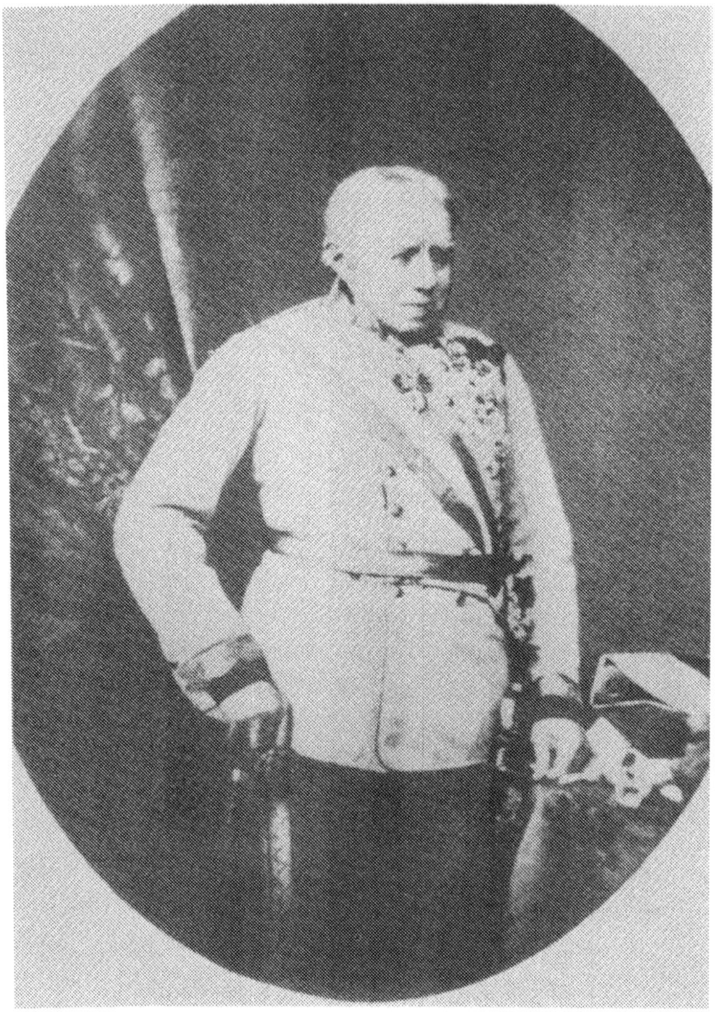

Fig. 5. Radetzky in 1857 (photo).

1850 an explanatory letter to Florent Cunier, the chief editor of the Annales d'oculistique in Brussels. The letter appeared in a French translation (by Binard)[17]. In it, Flarer reproduced verbatim a letter he had written in January 1841 to his friend, F. Jaeger in Vienna, in which he minutely describes the Field Marshall's condition, diagnosing it as a cancer with poor prognosis. Flarer complained bitterly about Hartung's behavior.

Cunier [18] added an epilogue in which he explained the diagnostic error

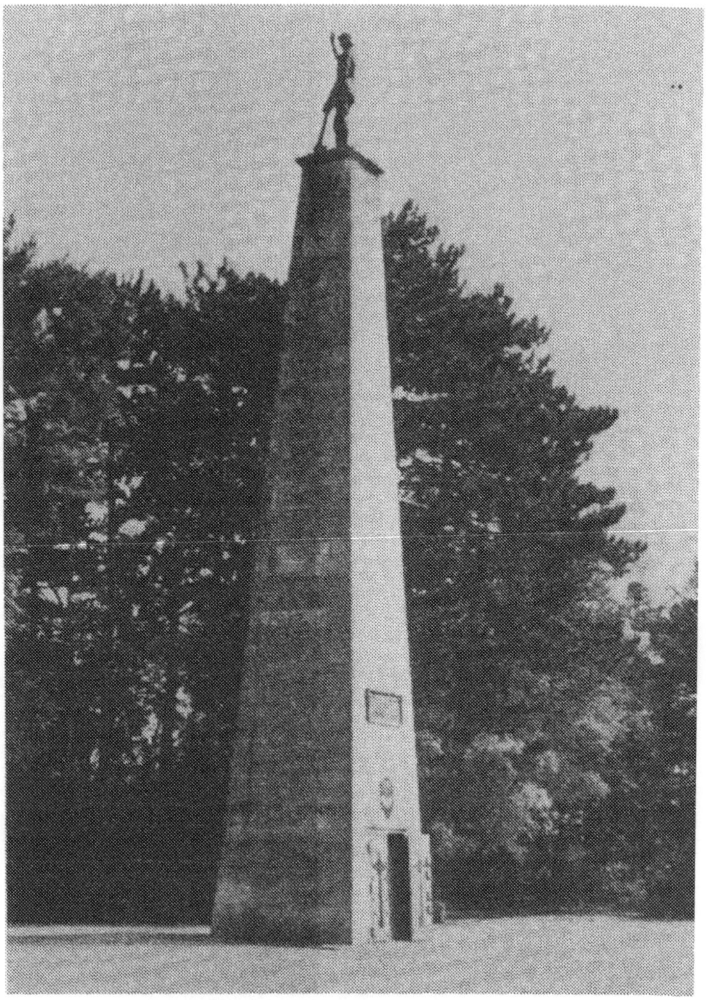

Fig. 6. Radetzky's tomb near Klein-Wetzdorf.

committed by Flarer and Jaeger and called them justified. He assumed it was an orbital abscess, a rare condition which should be reported whenever it is observed.

Friedrich *Jaeger* (1784–1871)[19] who was Beer's pupil and son-in-law, was seriously affected by this episode. In 1825 he had been appointed professor of ophthalmology at the Imperial Royal Medical-Surgical Joseph's Academy where he remained until 1848. He was at his time the greatest cataract surgeon in Europe and introduced the superior limbal

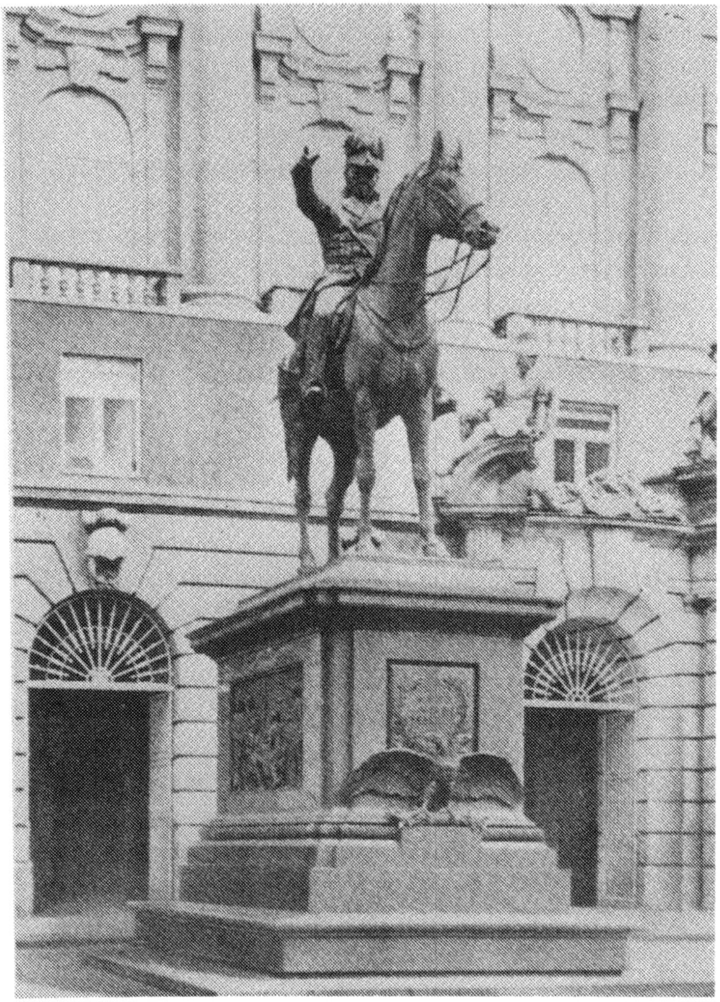

Fig. 7. The Radetzky monument by Kaspar von Zumbusch.

incision for the extraction. He was knighted by the emperor and became the personal physician and friend of prince and princess Metternich and of many diplomats and potentates. His three most famous pupils were A. v. Graefe, J. Sichel and his son, Eduard.

Jaeger had two great disappointments in his life. The first one was the cataract operation on Crown Prince Georg of Hannover. He performed the operation against his better judgment and the prince, the future King Georg V, remained blind.

The second was his error in diagnosing Radetzky's orbital tumefaction in 1841. Jaeger never quite recovered from this blow. In 1843 he published his version of the events [20]. He set the record straight and emphasized that the Field Marshall wanted only Dr. Hartung to treat him and only homeopathic medications to be administered.

Jaeger wrote a nearly identical statement to F. Cunier who read it in French [21] before a meeting of the Royal Belgian Academy of Medicine [22].

Jaeger's obituaries all allude to the unfortunate chain of events. Preyss [23] believed that it undermined his self-confidence and De Wecker [24] stated that Jaeger's unlucky period of life started 1839 with his operation on the crown prince of Hanover and ended in 1848 with the dissolution of the Josephinum. From then on he only worked in his private office with his son, Eduard.

The diagnosis

Only one factor is certain: the lesion in the Field Marshall's right orbit was not a neoplasm.

The history, clinical course and outcome would all speak for an orbital abscess secondary to an ethmoiditis. This is exactly the diagnosis suggested by De Wecker [24].

Some authors believe that Radetzky represents the first reported case of an orbital pseudotumor. Actually, this occurred nearly 1200 years earlier [25] and is described in chapter XXXII of an ecclesiastical history dealing "of one who was cured of a distemper in his eye at the relics of St. Cuthbert, A.D. 698." The clinical picture (swelling of the lids, unilateral exophthalmus, symptoms of inflammation, transient character) is that of an orbital inflammation.

Birch-Hirschfeld [26] in his monumental book on the orbit classifies Radetzky's case as belonging to group I of what he called orbital pseudotumors. Group I were orbital lesions, either infectious or inflammatory, which like all other groups clinically mimicked an orbital neoplasm. The term "orbital pseudotumor' has since then been generally accepted for orbital inflammations which clinically resemble an orbital neoplasm. Before Birch-Hirschfeld, the term "pseudoplasm" [27] was used though most authors implied a luetic infection. Occasional case reports in the Spanish literature [28] referred to orbital pseudotumor as unclassified non-neoplastic orbital lesions.

References

1. Hartung Chr. Krankheitsgeschichte Sr. Excellenz. des Herrn Feldmarschalls Grafen von Radetzky: Allgemeine homoeopathische Zeitung 20, issues 10 and 11, pages 145 and 161, 1841 (translated by Petroz and Roth in Annales d'ocul. 14: 164, 1845).
2. Kriegsarchiv - Hofkriegsrat 1841, 6, 5/2.
3. Griesselich L. War das eine Heilung mit sogenannten "Dezillionen"? Hygea, Zeitschrift besonders für rationell-specifische Heilkunst XV, issue 3, 1841 (translated in Annales d'ocul. 14: 174, 1954; abstracted in Schmidt's Jahrbücher der in– und ausländischen gesammten Medicin 34: 21, 1842, #283).
4. Anonymous. Eines Homeopathen Bassess: Allgemeine Zeitung für Chirurgie, innere Heilkunde und ihre Hilfswissenschaften II, issue 6, p. 51, February 5, 1842.
5. Anonymous. Untersuchung ueber die homeopathische Heilung eines Augenfungus; Allgemeine Zeitung für Chirurgie, innere Heilkunde und ihre Hilfswissenschaften II, issue 7, 1842 (abstracted in Schmidt's Jahrbücher der in- und ausländischen gesammten Medicin 34: 92, 1842, #358).
6. Anonymous: Geschichte und Documente der Heilung Sr. Exc. des k. k. Feldmarschalles etc. Grafen von Radetzky auf homeopathischen Wege gegenüber den Lügen und Schmähungen Pseudonymer; Dr. C. Wolfsche Buchdruckerei München 1843.
7. Cunier F. La vérité sur la guérison homéopathique de la maladie oculaire du Feld-Maréchal Autrichien Conte de Radetzky, Annales d'ocul. 23: 3, 1850.
8. Cartier. Bull. de l'Académie royale de Médecine de Belgique VIII: 263, 1849.
9. Fallot. Bull. de l'Académie royale de médecine de Belgique VIII: 1161, 1849.
10. Varlez. Bull. de l'Académie royale de médecine de Belgique IX: 262, 1850.
11. Fallot. Annales d'ocul. 23: 10, 1850.
12. Regele O. Feldmarschall Radetzky; Herold, Wien und München 1957.
13. Herre F. Radetzky: Kiepenhauer und Witsch. Köln 1981.
14. Grillparzer F. Feldmarschall Radetzky, in: Konstitutionelle Donauzeitung, June 1848 (in: Grillparzers sämtliche Werke, 5th edition, vol. I, pt. 2, p. 136; Cotta'sche Buchhandlung, Stuttgart 1893).
15. Hartung v. Hartungen KD. Mailänder Impressionen; Christoph Hartung und seine Beziehungen zu Radetzky und Hahnemann; Allgemeine homoeopath. Zeitung 213: 257, 1968.
16. Hirschberg J. The History of Ophthalmology (translated by FC Blodi); vol. 8b, p. 233, J.P. Wayenborgh, Bonn 1988.
17. Flarer F. Note sur la maladie oculaire du maréchal Radetzky; Annales d'ocul. 24: 23, 1850.
18. Cunier F. Epilogue; Annales d'ocul. 24: 29, 1850.
19. Hirschberg J. The History of Ophthalmology (translated by FC Blodi); vol. 5, p. 127, J.P. Wayenborgh, Bonn 1985.
20. Jaeger F. Et Audiatur altera pars; Hygea, Zeitschrift besonders für rationell-specifische Heilkunst XVIII: 158, 1843.
21. Cunier F. Communication relative à la guérison homoéopathique de la maladie oculaire de M. le maréchal Radetzky; Annales d'ocul. 23: 14, 1850.
22. Cunier F. Bull. de l'Académie royale de médecine de Belgique IX: 271, 1850.
23. Preyss v. Prof. Dr. Friedr. Jaeger Ritter v. Jaxthal; Wiener med. Presse 18: 1456, 1877.
24. De Wecker L. Frédéric Jaeger, chevalier de Jaxthal; Annales d'ocul. 69: 85, 1873.
25. The Venerable Bede. The Ecclesiastical History of the English Nation, p. 223; J.M. Dent and Sons, London and Toronto 1910.
26. Birch-Hirschfeld A. Krankheiten der Orbita; in: Graefe-Saemisch Handbuch der gesamten Augenheilkunde; second edition, IX/1/p. 500; Julius Springer, Berlin 1930.
27. Panas A. Des pseudoplasmes de l'orbite; Arch. d'opht. XV: 529, 1895.
28. Isola F. Pseudotumor orbitario; An. de oftalmologia (Mexico) VII: 3, 1904.

Documenta Ophthalmologica 71: 221–228, 1989.

The history of the ophthalmoscope

SPENCER E. SHERMAN
Department of Ophthalmology, Mount Sinai School of Medicine, 166 East 63rd Str., New York, NY 10021, USA

If one were living in 1849 and suffered a central retinal artery occlusion and were examined by the most eminent ophthalmologist of the day, the only diagnosis could be amaurosis or amblyopia. Why? Because visualization of the retina in vivo was still one year away.

There had been attempts to visualize the retina before 1850. In 1823, Purkinje from Czechoslovakia, constructed a crude model of an ophthalmoscope and seemed to solve the principles of imaging and illumination. However, his dissertation was in Latin and his audience was not receptive. He also did not grasp the impact of the moment. Therefore, the invention went by the wayside.

In 1845 Kussmaul from Germany seemed to solve the principle of imaging, but not that of illumination. In 1846, simultaneously, Cumming in England and Brücke in Germany solved the principle of illumination, but not that of imaging.

There were three principles that had to be solved in order to invent the ophthalmoscope. The first was that the patient and the observer had to be made emetropic, so that a point of focus on the retina of the patient would emanate from the eye in parallel rays of light and fall into focus on the retina of the observer. Secondly, the retina of the patient had to be sufficiently illuminated. And, thirdly, there had to be an optical alignment of the light source and the observer's pupil. These three principles were met by the imagination and creativity of Hermann von Helmholtz who, in 1851, to the Berlin Physical Society, presented his now famous and classic monograph, *Augenspiegel*, which in French meant ophthalmoscope, and in English meant eye speculum.

He invented the first monocular, reflecting, direct ophthalmoscope which produced an image which was virtual, erect, having a large magnification and a small field.

His ophthalmoscope consisted of superimposed glass plates which were simple, uncoated and held at an oblique angle to the light. The ophthalmoscope also had loose corrective concave lenses to correct the ametropia of the patient and the observer.

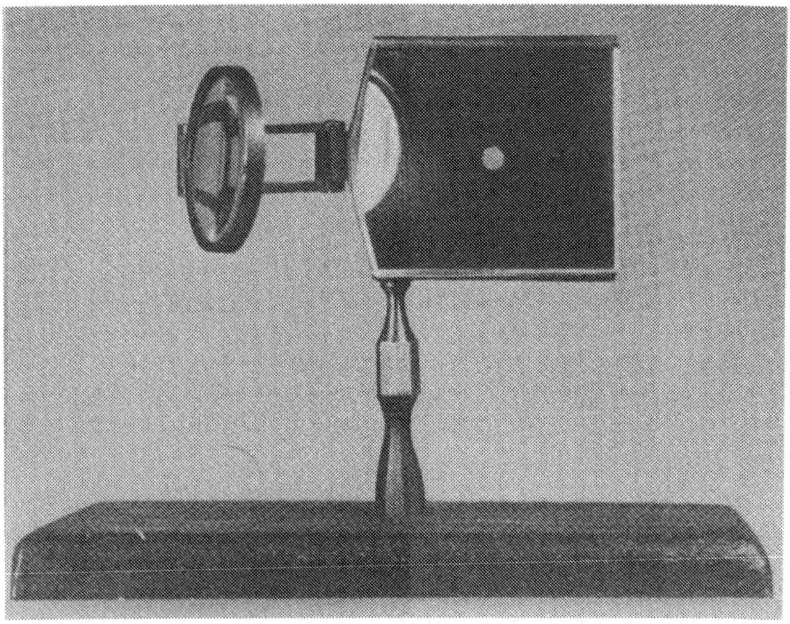

Fig. 1. A Coccius ophthalmoscope with lens clip and condensing lens. (Source: The Heidelberg Ophthalmic Museum.)

The superimposed glass plates were simultaneously reflective and transparent.

After von Helmholtz there have been thousands of ophthalmoscopes, mostly minor modifications of major innovations. The major innovations could be divided into two categories: 1) illumination and 2) reflecting surfaces. The quality of illumination progressed from the light of a candle to that of oil, then to that of gas and finally to electricity. The quality of the reflecting surface progressed from the superimposed glass plates of von Helmholtz to mirrors, both glass and metal, and then to a solid glass prism.

The first significant innovation in the development of the ophthalmoscope after von Helmholtz was by Epkens from Amsterdam who, in 1851, substituted a square plane glass mirror with a central opening for the superimposed glass plates of von Helmholtz.

The second important improvement was by von Helmholtz's instrument maker, Rekoss, who in 1852, from Germany, took the loose concave lenses which were used to correct the ametropia of the patient and observer and placed them into two disks, forever called "Rekoss' Disks" and are still used in the present day ophthalmoscope.

The next important modification was by Ruete in 1852 from Germany.

He utilized two biconvex condensing lenses in uprights in order to visualize the retina. He also substituted a concave mirror with a central opening for Epkens' square mirror. Ruete was the first to employ indirect ophthalmoscopy which produced a real but inverted image at the focal point of the condensing lens. The image was of small magnification but of large field.

In 1853 Coccius from Leipzig, Germany, produced three significant improvements of the ophthalmoscope. The first employed a square plane glass mirror with a central opening, and a biconvex condensing lens attached to the handle. Secondly, he added a lens clip for the observer in order to correct the ametropia. The third ophthalmoscope consisted of a round concave mirror with a central opening and a bar of lenses on the back of the ophthalmoscope for the observer in order to correct the ametropia (Fig. 1).

In 1854 Zehender, from Germany, substituted a metal convex mirror for the concave mirror plus a lens clip and also used a biconvex condensing lens for direct and indirect ophthalmoscopy (Fig. 2).

Ulrich, from Germany, in 1853 was the first to use tubes in the ophthalmoscope. One tube consisted of mirrors and lenses for the observer, and the

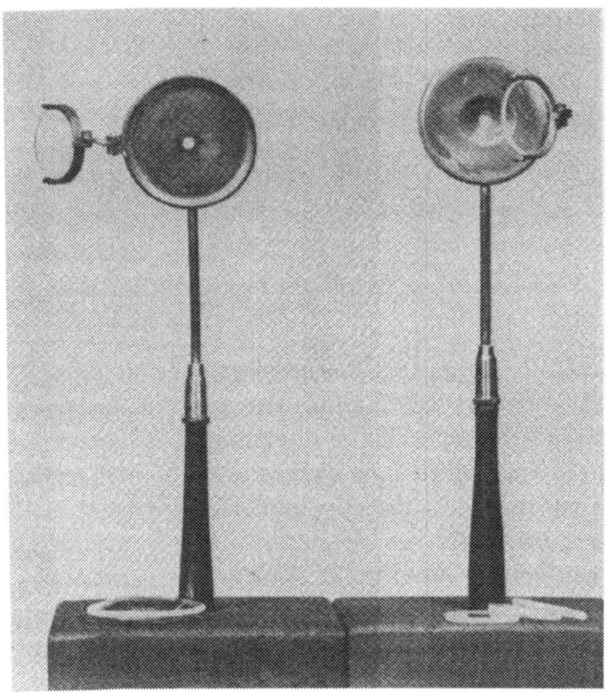

Fig. 2. A Zehender ophthalmoscope. Source: The Heidelberg Ophthalmic Museum.

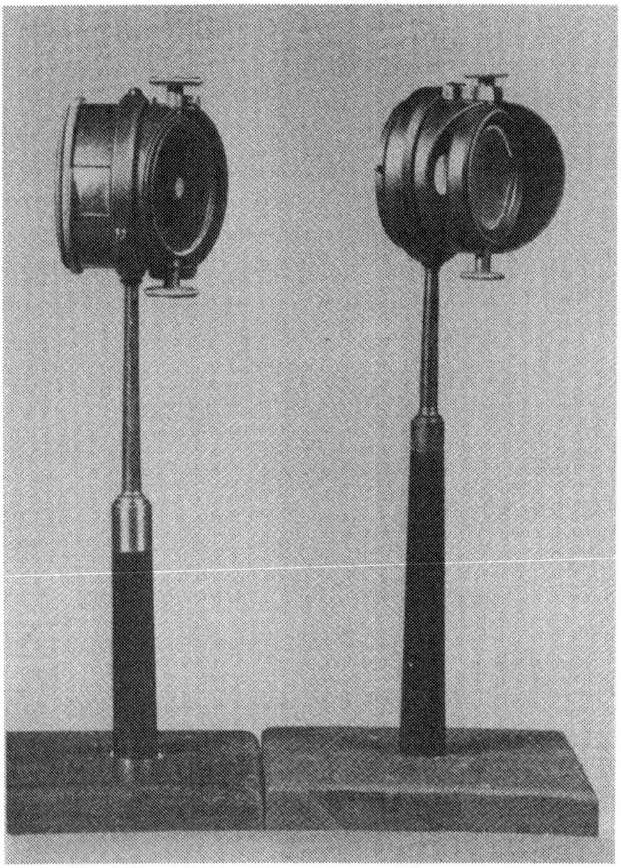

Fig. 3. The Jaeger ophthalmoscope. Source: The Heidelberg Ophthalmic Museum.

other tube was used to transmit light. The tubes were united at 40° and the method of ophthalmoscopy was that of indirect ophthalmoscopy.

In 1854, from Austria, Stellwag von Carion attached a concave nmirror to the handle of the ophthalmoscope by means of a joint. This was the first time that the mirror in ophthalmoscopy could be tilted.

Eduard Jaeger from Austria, in 1854, was the first to use interchangeable mirrors in the ophthalmoscope (Fig. 3). A plane mirror was used for direct ophthalmoscopy and a concave mirror plus a biconvex condensing lens was used for indirect ophthalmoscopy. Jaeger was also the first to measure refractive errors of the patient by means of the ophthalmoscope.

Richard Liebreich from Germany, in 1855, produced two significant ophthalmoscopes. The first was a large tubular ophthalmoscope with two

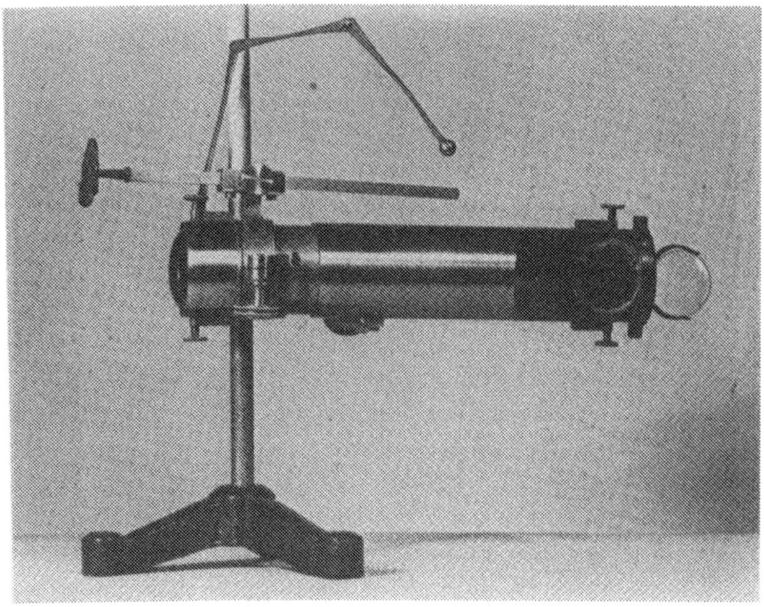

Fig. 4. A Liebreich ophthalmoscope. Source: The Heidelberg Ophthalmic Museum.

telescope tubes. One tube at the observer's end consisted of a concave moveable mirror while the other tube at the patient's end consisted of a concave lens. If one substituted a camera for the eye of the observer, this permitted photography of the retina. His second and much more popular ophthalmoscope was Liebreich's small portable ophthalmoscope which persisted for many decades. It consisted of a concave metal or glass mirror with a bevelled opening and an observer clip for lenses to correct the ametropia. It could be used for direct ophthalmoscopy or, with a biconvex condensing lens, for indirect ophthalmoscopy (Fig. 4).

The first ophthalmologist from the United States to improve upon the ophthalmoscope was Edward Loring from New York who, in 1869, invented three models of the ophthalmoscope. The first model was the so called "De Wecker" model. It consisted of detachable disks, one of convex lenses and the other of concave lenses. The second model had one disk of two rows of 23 lenses. The third model employed a mirror that could be tilted on the back of the ophthalmoscope plus a supplementary quadrant of lenses.

In 1883 John Couper from London invented an ophthalmoscope which was in the form of a magazine of loose lenses in a groove which could slide back and forth. This was improved upon by Morton from London in 1883, who mounted 29 lenses separately in an endless chain. The ophthalmoscope consisted of three disks, one disk for pupillary size, one disk consisting of a supplementary quadrant of lenses and the third disk which rotated the 29 lenses.

Although Edison invented the electric light bulb in 1878, it took seven more years to invent the first electric ophthalmoscope. This was accomplished by Dennett from New York who, in 1885, placed a small electric light bulb in the middle of the hollow handle of the ophthalmoscope. The wires from the ophthalmoscope were then attached to a dry cell battery.

Henry Juler, a famous maker of the ophthalmoscope from London, in 1886, improved upon the electric ophthalmoscope. He placed the electric light bulb on the outside of the handle just below the mirror.

Charles May from New York in 1900 invented two ophthalmoscopes, of which the first consisted of two disks of concave and convex lenses. His most significant innovation in the ophthalmoscope was the substitution of a solid glass prism for the mirror in 1914. This ophthalmoscope could run both by battery and electricity. The reflections and distortions of mirrors had been a problem during the early days of the invention of the ophthalmoscope. The mirrors were improved upon by Marple from New York in 1906 who invented a "U" shaped mirror. De Zeng from New Jersey in 1907 placed a notch in the mirror and, of course, Charles May in 1914, substituted the solid glass prism for the mirror.

If one now considers binocular ophthalmoscopes, one has to return to Paris in 1861 where Giraud Teulon invented the first binocular indirect ophthalmoscope (Fig. 5). It consisted of a large concave mirror and two glass prisms. Using a biconvex condensing lens he was able to visualize the retina by indirect ophthalmoscopy. The binocular ophthalmoscope was improved upon by Charles Schepens from Belgium, in 1946. He invented the first electric binocular indirect ophthalmoscope that is presently being used in today's ophthalmoscopy.

Later developments in the ophthalmoscope have been as follows: 1) a battery in the handle of the ophthalmoscope for a truly portable ophthalmoscope; 2) the giant scope for greater visualization of the retina; 3) a rechargeable ophthalmoscope; and 4) a halogen light bulb for improved illumination.

Thus we can see that even one decade after the invention of the ophthalmoscope the world of diagnosis was opened not only to ophthalmology but to all of medicine. For instance, in 1853 Donders discovered pigmentary retinopathy. In 1853 Coccius visualized the retina and could see a retinal detachment in vivo for the first time. In 1855, von Graefe discoverd the cupped disc in glaucoma and in the same year Liebreich visualized a central

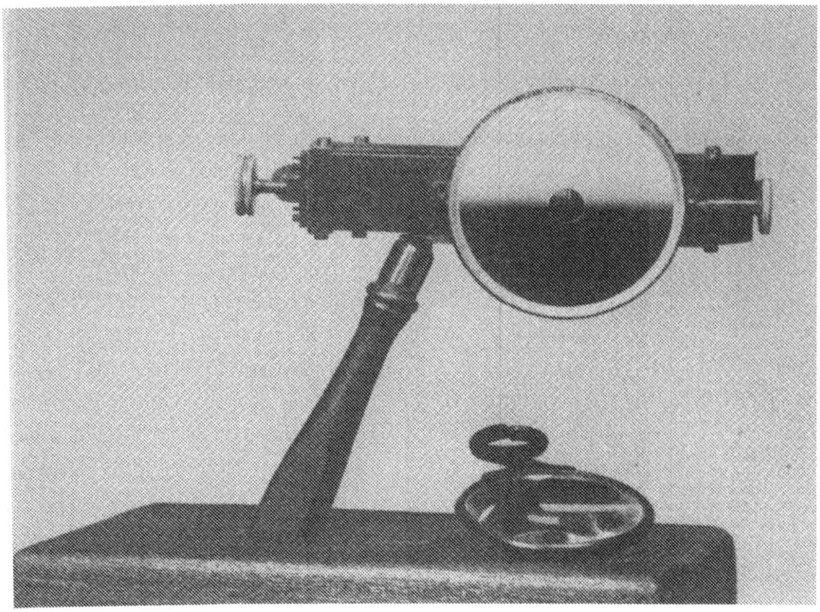

Fig. 5. The Giraud-Teulon binocular indirect ophthalmoscope. Source: The Heidelberg Ophthalmic Museum.

retinal thrombosis. In 1856 Heyman discovered hypertensive retinopathy in the eye, and in 1858 Jacobson visualized syphilitic retinitis. In 1860 von Graefe discovered papilledema, and in 1861 Jaeger noted optic atrophy.

References

1. Allbrett T. On the use of the ophthalmoscope. New York: MacMillan & Co., 1871; 13–21.
2. Angell H. A treatise on diseases of the eye. Boston: Jane Campbell, 1870; 18–32.
3. Fuchs E. Text-book of ophthalmology. New York: D. Appleton & Co., 1892; 1–14.
4. Helmholtz H. Beschreibung eines Augenspiegels zur Untersuchung der Netzhaut im lebenden Auge. Berlin, 1851.
5. Jacobson E. Diseases of the eye. New York: W.B. Saunders, 1899; 78–103.
6. Laurence I. A handy book of ophthalmic surgery. Philadelphia: Henry Lea, 1869; 2–29.
7. Loring E. Text-book of ophthalmoscopy. New York: D. Appleton & Co., 1896; 1–20.
8. May C. Manual of the diseases of the eye. New York: William Wood & Co., 1900; 1834.
9. Mittendorf W. A manual on diseases of the eye and ear. New York: G.P. Putnam & Sons, 1881; 228–38.
10. Parsons J. Diseases of the eye. London: J & A Churchill, 1907; 114–44.
11. Rucker WC. A history of the ophthalmoscope. Rochester, Minnesota: Whiting Printers and Stationers, 1977; 127.
12. Schmidt-Rimpler H. Ophthalmology and Ophthalmoscopy. New York: William Wood & Co., 1884; 3–11.

13. Schett A. St. Gallen, Switzerland, personal communication.
14. Shosted TH. The description of an ophthalmoscope. Chicago: Cleveland Press, 1916; 7–33.
15. Swanzy H. A handbook of the diseases of the eye. Philadelphia: Blakiston's Son & Co., 1898; 77–89.
16. Thornington J. The ophthalmoscope and how to use it. Philadelphia: Blakiston's Son & Co., 1906; 1–43.

www.ingramcontent.com/pod-product-compliance
Ingram Content Group UK Ltd.
Pitfield, Milton Keynes, MK11 3LW, UK
UKHW020239160926
475610UK00001B/62
9780792302735